BEYOND LONGEVITY

Hay House Titles of Related Interest

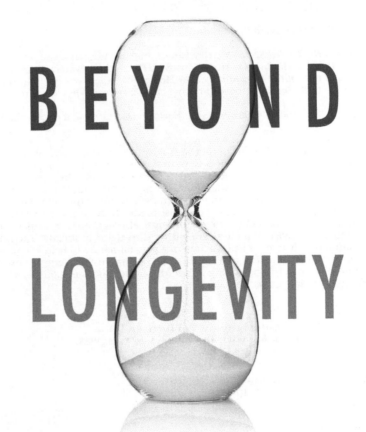

BEYOND LONGEVITY

A Proven Plan for Healing Faster,
Feeling Better, and Thriving at Any Age

JASON PRALL

HAY HOUSE, INC.
Carlsbad, California • New York City
London • Sydney • New Delhi

Copyright © 2022 by Jason Prall

Published in the United States by: Hay House, Inc.: www.hayhouse.com®
Published in Australia by: Hay House Australia Pty. Ltd.: www.hayhouse.com.au
Published in the United Kingdom by: Hay House UK, Ltd.: www.hayhouse.co.uk
Published in India by: Hay House Publishers India: www.hayhouse.co.in

Cover design: Milan Bozic • *Interior design:* Karim J. Garcia • *Indexer:* Joan Shapiro

**Cataloging-in-Publication Data
is on file with the Library of Congress**

Hardcover ISBN: 978-1-4019-5839-8
E-book ISBN: 978-1-4019-5840-4
Audiobook ISBN: 978-1-4019-5842-8

10 9 8 7 6 5 4 3 2 1
1st edition, December 2022

Printed in the United States of America

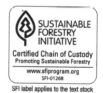

SUSTAINABLE FORESTRY INITIATIVE
Certified Chain of Custody
Promoting Sustainable Forestry
www.sfiprogram.org
SFI-01268

SFI label applies to the text stock

This book is dedicated to my Mother.
Thank you for your tremendous sacrifice,
unwavering support, and dedication to
always putting your family first.

CONTENTS

LETTER TO THE READER

In my 20 years of investigating the human condition, I've come to realize that our potential for health is inherent within us. Health is not created by a doctor, device, or anything external. This is worth repeating . . .

Your health potential is *inherent to your being*.

Life is a mysterious process with a natural development, order, and cycle. It is lent to us for a brief moment before the physical body is left behind. If we want to thrive in the modern world, preserve health, and strive for *more than* longevity, we must create a mental, emotional, physical, and energetic environment that is congruent with this natural lifecycle.

This book combines the knowledge from my own personal experience with that of Western scientific research, Ayurvedic wisdom, and over 100 health experts, along with the wisdom of more than 30 amazing elders around the planet I met while filming *The Human Longevity Project* docuseries. I encourage you to also visit www.beyondlongevitybook.com for a deeper dive into the studies and research that form the foundation of this book. When experiential wisdom is supported by the latest scientific research, a more integrated picture emerges of how you can most effectively increase your happiness, health, and longevity.

— Jason Prall

INTRODUCTION

DISCOVERING HEALTH

On the basketball court at 13 years old is where my chronic knee pain began. What appeared to be a minor, acute injury at the time unfolded into a 20-year struggle that bounced me around from doctors and physical therapists to orthopedic surgeons and rehab specialists. When rest and ice didn't work, strengthening exercises and pain medications were offered as solutions. When exercise therapy didn't work, surgery was recommended. After slicing through my patellar tendon and scraping out clusters of calcified deposits and scar tissue from my knee, four months of rest and rehab awaited me, only for the pain to return within a year. In my early 20s, I learned to accept that chronic knee pain was just going to be part of my life going forward.

Not long after, I came face-to-face with my next challenge, as I was diagnosed with a facial skin condition known as seborrheic dermatitis. Again, I looked to the trusted professionals for a solution. Despite the protocols and prescriptions from credentialed specialists, I was continually plagued with itchy, scaly, and oily patches on my face that would regularly peel off from forehead to chin—leaving tender, freshly exposed dermal layers that gave my face a warm pink glow as if I was just pulled out of the oven.

This was the moment I began to give up on the traditional Western medical system. The solutions I was given for seemingly straightforward chronic conditions proved absolutely worthless. And in the case of my skin condition, the prescriptions made things worse. Just 21 years old, with scant resources beyond my keyboard and an antiquated WebCrawler search engine, I took it upon myself to find the solution.

As a broke college kid with a part-time job, I was unable to afford any "alternative" doctors outside of the coverage provided by my health insurance. To find solutions I could practically attempt, I plunged down endless rabbit holes in search of answers. As I implemented therapies and techniques that intuitively felt right, it became clear that there was no single cause nor single solution to my conditions. Approaching a singular aspect of health would reveal another interconnected issue, like peeling the layers of an onion. I would need to heal on multiple levels to get to the core of my issues. I couldn't just address the pain in my knee or a patch of skin; I needed to make fundamental lifestyle changes. This experience challenged every programmed belief I had about health and taught me how to think about personalized medicine.

CALLED TO THE HEALING PATH

With the goal of empowering those suffering a similar fate and the dire need by so many, I felt a strong call to walk the healing path. In 2012, I made the decision to leave my 10-year mechanical engineering career behind to start my private integrative health practice.

In many ways, the skills required to be a successful engineer translate quite well to the health world. What drew me to engineering to begin with was my natural tendency and ability to use a systems-thinking approach to complex problems. Understanding how individual parts interact with one another and affect the system as a whole is a necessary skill if you're working on airplane design, a building's heating system, *and* when analyzing dysfunction in the body. To be successful in the field of integrative and holistic health, systems thinking is absolutely essential.

In order to execute high-level research in areas such as social genomics, emotional trauma, immunology, mitochondrial medicine, happiness, and metabolomics, the specialists involved tend to be narrowly focused on a given topic of expertise. Too often, these experts end up in intellectual silos and have little incentive or ability to engage in cross-disciplinary study and interaction. Approaching the idea of human health with a natural inclination for systems thinking, I was able to see how typically compartmentalized areas of research fit together to impact the health of an individual. My unique perspective allowed me to extract the practical wisdom and identify the most important factors that encourage health, which I discuss in this book.

As I crossed paths withan increasing number of integrative health practitioners, they shared similar stories. Many of these doctors who became my teachers and mentors were spurred into a more functional or integrative practice because they were unable to resolve their own health challenges or those of their patients using a traditional Western medical model. Their research led them beyond simple diagnostics, medication, and surgery, and I fell in love with this nuanced and holistic approach.

Through years of self-study, functional and integrative coursework, certifications, and advanced training by experienced medical professionals, my work as an integrative health practitioner began taking shape. Despite my lack of standard medical credentials, I was able to build my credentials through a variety of functional practitioner courses, seminars, and trainings with some of the most respected functional medicine and ayurvedic clinicians in the world. This gave me the tools to be able to work with clients suffering from some of the most complex cases of autoimmune conditions, food sensitivities, hormonal imbalances, sleep disturbances, infections, chronic gastrointestinal disorders, thyroid conditions, chronic fatigue, and unspecified symptoms and syndromes. But no matter how much research I read, how many courses I took, or how well I memorized biological pathways, none of that knowledge compared with the wisdom I gained working in depth with clients one-on-one. These individuals became my greatest teachers because we were able to go deep into their health history, physical ailments, emotional framework, mindset, and lifestyle practices. And over time I realized that, for a doctor or practitioner, this is where all the valuable information resides.

The Western medical system has made great strides toward healing a variety of conditions, oftentimes through mind-blowing advancements in technology. Still, many of the discussions on health and disease continue to push for solutions that disempower the individual: always more doctors, more pills, and more interventions. And yet, paradoxically, we have examples of very healthy people across the planet that are not only alive but thriving into old age without many of these proposed Western solutions. This recognition began to heavily influence my philosophy on health and eventually led me on a journey to learn firsthand from these fascinating people.

This investigation culminated in a nine-part documentary film series, *The Human Longevity Project*, which eventually reached hundreds of thousands of viewers. The incredible exploration took me across the globe to gather knowledge and wisdom from dozens of elders and the most respected health experts on the planet from numerous scientific fields, including gerontology, antiaging medicine, nutrition, immunology, functional medicine, social genomics, food science, chronobiology, toxicology, genetics, microbiology, neurology, and bioinformatics. I was also fortunate to speak with a variety of experts in areas of children's health, emotional trauma, environmental health, biophysics, mitochondrial science, herbal medicine, bioenergetics, biohacking, mental health, and emotional well-being.

MEETING THE ELDERS

Over the course of 14 months, filmmaker John Dahlgren and I set out to interview dozens of individuals who were healthy well into their 80s, 90s, and beyond 100. We would come to refer to them collectively as "the elders" because of their wide age ranges and the immense wisdom they would impart throughout our journey. Our goal was to learn not just about how they live today but also about their environment and lifestyle from a historical perspective. And, more importantly to me, I wanted to examine their health through the lens of the latest scientific research, beyond the simple correlation studies and genetic theories. I sought to identify how, biologically speaking, their environment, lifestyle, and behavior might actually translate to healthy aging.

In order to find this diverse group of individuals from a variety of cultures who could share their wisdom with us, we began our search in the "blue zones." These identified regions are based on the work of demographer Michel Poulain who, after years of field study, first identified and confirmed that a tiny, mountainous region on the island of Sardinia, Italy, had an extraordinary number of people living beyond 100 years of age. According to Michel, he circled this mountainous region on a map and shaded it with a blue pen, dubbing it the first blue zone. Later, Michel teamed up with author Dan Buettner and National Geographic to identify more regions that met their statistical criteria for exceptional longevity. They included Okinawa, Japan; Ikaria, Greece; Loma Linda, California, in the United States; and Nicoya, Costa Rica. However, our focus wasn't on identifying what was special about a particular geographical location, but instead asking what we could learn from these elders that would be meaningful to someone living in a modern, industrialized society.

Before we could answer this question, we would have to find a collection of elders who would be willing to donate their most valuable commodity—their precious time. Unfortunately there is no public registry identifying the names, locations, and e-mail addresses of centenarians. We couldn't just call or e-mail them to set up an interview. So we honed our search to small village settings and enlisted the help of "fixers" who could help us arrange meetings. The ideal fixer was somebody local, who spoke both English and the native language for purposes of translation, and who was familiar with the residents and their customs.

With the help of our fixers, John and I would often start by asking the village locals if they knew anybody over the age of 90 or 100. Our connections might begin with our Airbnb host, or perhaps the owner of a nearby health store, or the worker at the surf shop. They would often direct us to a villager who had been around for decades and knew everybody. Inevitably these connections would lead us to the door of a local elder we would hope to interview.

This was a fascinating, occasionally uncomfortable, and mostly enjoyable process. Frequently we would show up unannounced or with only a day's notice: a couple of Americans, a translator, and a mound of film equipment. In just about every instance, the family welcomed us in with open arms. Once we got to know them a bit, they seemed to relish the opportunity to share their culture, life story, and philosophy of healthy living—and usually with a heavy dose of humor sprinkled in. And as we wrapped up our interviews, they often insisted that we stay for a meal, perhaps some wine, and a few laughs. For John and me, there was a palpable sense of nostalgia, recalling our own roots in small towns and tight-knit communities in Washington state.

In Sardinia, we had the pleasure of getting to know Giulio, who at 104 still rode his bike every day. In Okinawa, we spent time with the amazing 97-year-old Hideko, who was still able to till her soil, read the newspaper without glasses, and, according to her daughter, was climbing her trees to harvest oranges until the age of 95. On the island of Ikaria, we drank tea with Orestis and laughed as he shared stories about his youth and reminded us that despite being 98 years old, he was still participating in the all-night village parties known as Panigiri.

A large subsection of longevity research continues to focus on the current lifestyle of elders and the regions that consistently produce them. They often want to know what they do, how they eat, how they move, and about their relationships. This is all well and good, but it is only a small part of the picture. We went further, asking what life was like growing up and how their parents raised them. We spoke with them at length about how the local lifestyles have changed over the years, how industry and technology have impacted their community, and about the current social issues regarding the way people live today. And, not least, we asked them what they think contributed to their exceptionally long and healthy life.

In short order, it became obvious that the historical context of their life painted a very different picture from the way locals are living today—a previous way of life that has all but vanished in these villages and has long been paved over by the same industry and technology we see in the Western world. It was such a rare gift to hear firsthand accounts of what life was like in 1930 Ikaria or 1940 Costa Rica. The process of giving birth, how children were raised, how food and water were sourced, the modes of transportation, how they dealt with infections or food shortages . . . it is almost unimaginable to fully comprehend a day in the life described to us by the elders. They had privileges and advantages we in the West no longer have the luxury of experiencing. They also faced hardships and daily struggles, the likes of which would make even the most hardened Westerner cringe.

THE SIMPLE LIFE

The elders we spoke with described their younger years as ones of profound simplicity. Tight-knit and often large families were the norm. And they relied heavily on their village networks for security, survival, and to minimize struggle. As young children, they often helped the family grow and harvest food. Most of the elders I got to know walked to school or to town for most of their life. And occasionally they might have taken a horse-drawn wagon for longer journeys, perhaps to a neighboring town to visit a relative.

That said, there can be a tendency to romanticize the simplicity and slower pace of these previous eras. But these elders lived no easy life. Many of them dealt with bouts of low food supply and famine. They had a strong work ethic and were willing to make great sacrifices. I'm reminded of a conversation with a 99-year-old man from the town of Villagrande in Sardinia. Michelino Scudu is as hilarious as he is energetic, always teasing and joking during our conversations. With a tone and delivery that was equal parts playful and stern, he asserted, "Young people today drive cars and walk too little. I used to walk to Tortolì, three hours on foot before hoeing the wheat fields, along with my wife. Then we came back home, my wife would start the dinner, peeled the potatoes, prepared the minestrone while I was reading the paper. And if the man would deserve the Nobel Prize, I think the woman would have deserved a double Nobel Prize for the same reason. Women are very hardworking, especially older women. Our mothers sacrificed themselves to raise us and form a family. Young people don't work hard enough nowadays. We used to do a very hard job and we walked a lot. Today everyone just drives everywhere. They are born driving a car. We were born in the dust," followed by a burst of laughter.

It's a difficult task to truly recognize how much technology has changed the way we operate. Still, almost a century ago, the industrialized world was already using automobiles, electricity, refrigeration, and commercial air travel. Over the next 30 years, industrialized societies witnessed monumental growth in technology, and convenience exploded. Not so for the residents of the rural villages we interviewed in Okinawa, Nicoya, Sardinia, and Ikaria—they didn't get electricity until the 1960s or '70s. This meant no refrigerators or freezers. They didn't have cars, televisions, radios, light bulbs, phones, computers, automatic dishwashers, microwaves, electric ovens, washers, or dryers for much of their life. Many didn't have indoor plumbing. Drinking water usually came from a spring or a well, not from a city water supply. Homes, if they had heat, were warmed by a fireplace or woodburning stove. Food was grown, foraged, raised, and hunted by family and friends. And because of slow and expensive distribution systems, any food that was brought in usually consisted of only staples such as coffee, tea, spices, and sugar. This lifestyle was not much of a choice—it reflected the resources they had, the unique environmental conditions, and the ways of their ancestors. It was all they knew.

Just about everything we rely on in the modern, industrialized world was nonexistent. Despite the struggle and demanding work, comfort and convenience were not a priority nor a core value. This fostered a completely different mindset than we see today in Western cultures. A life lived in simplicity, close to nature, and in the tight community appeared to cultivate humility, connection, and gratitude. Meals were eaten together, and evenings were passed in conversation with friends and neighbors. They didn't take things for granted like so many of us do in the modern world. "It was important to be fulfilled and happy with your belongings. So I never said, 'the other person has more.' Whatever God gives me, I am happy with it," said Yannoula Kratzas from Ikaria.

None of the elders in the villages we visited had practical access to a medical system for most of their lives. Instead, they were forced to rely on folk remedies passed down through the generations. Their medicine consisted of herbal connections, teas, salves, foods, and a lot of wisdom. They are living proof that high-tech medical advances, while exciting and mostly helpful for a variety of conditions, are not *required* to remain healthy as we age. If anything, the elders show us the tremendous value of simplifying our approach to life when possible. They were adamant that it was their simple lifestyle and a shared understanding of how to harmonize with their respective environments that led to exceptional mental, emotional, and physical well-being.

A MODERN-AGE PARADOX

Even though our film series was called *The Human Longevity Project*, one of the things that became most clear after visiting with dozens of elders around the world was that it wasn't only about how many years were in your life (your lifespan), but how much life was in your years (your health span). It is common to view the concept of longevity as an ideal scenario where we maintain relatively good function until our last breath. But while the concept of longevity seems sexy, it's insufficient and hollow—what most of us really want is an extended life filled with vibrant health, meaning, and purpose. We want to *thrive* as we age. We dream of a life that is full of joy, connection, service, and new experiences, with a healthy curiosity of how the future will unfold.

The slow, natural rhythm and go-with-the-flow energy described by the elders provide a glaring juxtaposition to a fast-paced, technology-dependent, structured city life. The elders we met lived simply because they had to. They didn't have booming industry acting as a major fulcrum to yield an abundance of convenience and comfort. They tended to find more manual, natural, and often elegant solutions to life's demands. Not surprisingly, these solutions often reduced complexity, environmental pollution, unintended consequences, and long-term health issues for the community. Placing too much value on convenience and comfort unquestionably invites long-term health risk, increased dissatisfaction, and greater suffering.

And yet, we can't re-create the antiquated, 20th-century lifestyle of those who grew up in these longevity-rich environments. Their experiences come from a bygone era. There's no going back. The dominant culture is too entrenched in technology and convenience to return to an ultra-simple village life. And despite the challenges we've created for ourselves, I'm quite confident most wouldn't want to go back. As I listened to story after story from the elders, I was constantly reminded of how lucky I am to be living in such comfort. We can observe and learn from the elders, but we cannot expect society at large to replicate their path. If we are prudent, however, we can apply their lessons and wisdom to our modern world in novel ways. In ways that not only make room for technological advancement but also help shape the direction of technology and harmoniously guide the progress of society.

By cutting through the sentimental allure of the past, we can also adopt the best of what modern science reveals about health and longevity. That is the promise of this book—you will learn how to apply timeless and scientifically supported health wisdom to your life in many ways so you can heal faster and thrive as you age. In Part I, I'll outline a framework to illustrate the underlying fundamentals of life—*what* is biologicalical aging and how we heal. Then, in Part II, the focus is on the primary aspects of healthy living. I'll use a systems-thinking approach to connect the dots that most people miss between the latest science and the wisdom of the elders. It is important to understand, however, that this isn't a one-size-fits-all, cookie-cutter approach. My intent is to empower you with the necessary knowledge and understanding to implement only what makes sense in the context of your own circumstances.

Each day, we are presented with an opportunity to choose a more harmonious path that establishes greater coherence within ourselves, one another, and the environment. And when we live from alignment, all life benefits.

PART I

THE BUILDING BLOCKS OF LIFE

Chapter 1

THE SCIENCE OF AGING
AND LONGEVITY

Living matter evades the decay to equilibrium.

— Erwin Schrödinger

WHAT IS LIFE?

It's quite remarkable how easy it is to take for granted the miracle and mystery of life. What does it mean to be alive? Where does life reside in the physical body? Is there life in your elbow? And if you lose your arm, are you less alive? When does life begin? When does it end?

The more we think about it, the criteria for life is confusing, if nothing else. The complexity and magic behind human biology is mind-numbing. Despite decades of scientific research, we can't conclusively identify how every part works in isolation, let alone understand the dynamic interplay of all that makes us human. From conception, the body and mind respond and adapt to an immense range of environmental conditions, with near-infinite complexity in a seamless cosmic dance.

This leads to one of the fundamental questions biologists ask today. Who are we on the physical level? What does it mean to be human? Scientific understanding seems to point to the idea that each of us is an amazingly complex ecosystem of genetic lifeforms that communicate and coordinate activity in ways we still cannot grasp. It's been estimated that we have somewhere around 1 billion-*trillion* biochemical reactions happening every *second* inside the human body! So who or what is actually in charge of that biological activity? To answer this question, we'll explore three distinct sets of genomes that are essential for your life—your human genome, your mitochondrial genome, and your microbiome.

THE HUMAN GENOME

Of course we cannot neglect the status of your genome in our discussion of health and aging. Within your DNA (deoxyribonucleic acid) exists the entire blueprint for your unique human life. Just as the tiny acorn contains all the information it needs to grow into a mighty oak tree, your DNA contains all the information necessary to build, repair, and maintain your body.

An important part of this equation is RNA (ribonucleic acid), which is responsible for making copies of the DNA in order to produce new proteins and cells during growth or when the old cells and cellular parts need to be replaced. Ideally, this process happens without error. But the human genome is fragile. As damage occurs, there is a loss of genomic stability, and your DNA blueprint cannot be perfectly copied to produce new, unblemished cells and cellular parts. Like a Xerox copy, the quality of reproduction fades as you make a copy of a copy of a copy of a copy. As a result, we see loss of enzyme function, genetic base pair mutations, stem cell exhaustion, poor intracellular communication, mitochondrial dysfunction, and shortened telomeres. All of which continue to perpetuate a cycle of damage and dysfunction on the cellular level.

But here's the thing: your DNA also contains the necessary information to *repair* all sorts of damage. Telomerase—the enzyme that lengthens telomeres—is one such example. Telomeres are small bits of genetic code that reside at the end of chromosomes to protect them from damage and provide greater stability to the DNA. The longer the telomeres, the greater the protection to the DNA. Other repair mechanisms include processes such as nucleotide excision repair, base excision repair, mismatch repair, and DNA double strand break repair. Additionally, your cells have the capability to turn back the clock, so to speak. Cellular stress signals can activate a process of cellular de-differentiation, turning mature cells into immature ones by rewinding their developmental path, reaching the stem cell state. These immature cells can then re-differentiate in order to create healthy new cells, allowing organs and tissues to regenerate.

Again, it must be reiterated, that your DNA is merely the architectural plan. In order to execute various repair aspects of the blueprint, energetic signals are required to express necessary gene transcripts. So looking to the human genome alone for the answer to disease and aging is insufficient.

THE MITOCHONDRIAL GENOME

Next we have mitochondria, a common focal point in both chronic disease and longevity research. Located inside most cells, the average adult houses approximately 100 quadrillion of these tiny organelles in their body. They are primarily known as the "powerhouse" of the cell for their role in turning oxygen, nutrients, and food substrates into electricity, light, and ATP, which are the primary energy sources for the cell and body as a whole. In this way, they are like the cell's batteries and digestive system.

Mitochondria are responsible for much more than just energy generation. In the process of making energy, mitochondria also generate reactive oxygen species (ROS), also known as free radicals or oxidative stress, as a part of normal operation. They produce heat and release light as a byproduct of this energy generation. All these outputs—the ATP, ROS, heat, and light—act as signaling mechanisms that direct function both inside the cell and outside the cell. Mitochondria communicate directly with your cell nucleus and human DNA, assist in detoxification, synthesize hormones, and even regulate programmed cell death. In recent years, researchers have also begun to elucidate danger response signals and mechanisms that mitochondria use to communicate to other cells in the presence of pathogens and toxins. And all of this is merely a fraction of what they do.

With all this in mind, probably the most important factor when considering the role of mitochondria in the aging process is the fact that they have their own specialized, circular DNA that is completely distinct and independent from our helical human DNA located in the cell nucleus. This means we all have non-human DNA inside our cells working autonomously and symbiotically with our own human DNA to maintain healthy and balanced function at the cellular level. It should be no surprise then, as we look at the manifestation of all forms of chronic disease, indeed we also find significant damage to mitochondria and mitochondrial DNA. For example, if the function of pancreatic cell is to produce insulin, and mitochondrial damage in this pancreatic cell is significantly high, the cell may fail to adequately produce insulin—a hallmark characteristic of type 2 diabetes. As mitochondrial DNA mutations increase in a given cell, so does dysfunction and the presence of chronic disease symptoms. Without a doubt, mitochondria are central players in health and aging.

THE GENOME OF YOUR MICROBIOTA

The role of microbes in human health is undoubtedly the new, great frontier in biological research. Hundreds of millions of dollars are being dumped into research focused on how microbiota are related to various disease conditions such as heart disease, cancer, dementia, diabetes, autoimmune disease, skin conditions, and the like. Current estimates indicate the average adult consists of about 38 trillion bacterial cells and only about 30 trillion human cells. Added together, the microbes contain far more coding genes than does the human genome. One could argue that you are, in fact, more microbe than you are human. Yet none of the mainstream aging theories factor in the activity or role of microbiota.

The microorganisms that live on and in our bodies include bacteria, viruses, fungi, archaea, protozoa, and helminths. And they all appear to be carrying out important functions within the giant ecosystem that is the body. These microbiota are commonly associated with the gastrointestinal tract. (That's why you'll see so many products focused on getting so-called good bacteria, or probiotics, into your gut.) But truth is, you'll be hard-pressed to find anywhere in or on the body where microbiota don't exist. Researchers are finding them everywhere they look—in the mouth, eyes, brain, lungs, placenta, ovaries, uterus, bile ducts, urogenital tract, seminal fluid, in and on the skin, and of course in the gastrointestinal tract.

While an exact number is difficult to nail down, it's commonly estimated that microbes influence anywhere from 70 to 98 percent of your biological function. Brilliantly, your genetic code has outsourced most of the labor and function to the vast array of microbes living in and on your body, forming a truly symbiotic and co-dependent relationship. We are all immensely dependent on these microbes for healthy function.

WHAT IS AGING?

What is aging? Over the years, I've asked dozens of experts this question, including medical professionals, gerontologists, fitness experts, nutritionists, and academic researchers. Every single person has given a different answer, and few were alike. The most common response I received was, in joking fashion, that aging is essentially the process of getting older. Others mentioned loss of function and greater susceptibility to disease, while still others spoke of various mechanisms and cellular components such as mitochondria and telomeres.

There are four main characteristics of biological aging about which most aging and longevity scientists agree:

1. Aging is deleterious or harmful to the organism.
2. Aging is a progressive and ongoing process.
3. Aging is a built-in or inherent process to the organism.
4. Aging is universal to all living beings.

An adjacent, relevant characteristic is that the rate of aging is specific to each species. Interestingly, while we have this general consensus on the characteristics of aging, there isn't a consensus on what fundamentally drives the process of aging—let alone how to slow it down or "reverse" it.

Biomarkers to Measure Biological Age

Many researchers are attempting to identify a measurable human biomarker that accurately reflects the *biological* age of a person. The idea is that as an individual's saliva, blood, or urine gets tested, the estimated biological age based on the biomarker can be compared with the individual's actual chronological age.

For example, if a 60-year-old woman gets tested and her biomarker reflects that of the average 40-year-old woman, she could be classified as very healthy and biologically "younger" than her actual age. And, in theory, we should be able to predict how much life is ahead of her because she is aging slower on the biological level than the average woman born in the same year.

So far, the two most promising candidates for estimating biological age are known as the epigenetic clock and the bioenergetic clock. Epigenetic clocks pertain mostly to the DNA methylation status of a cell, while bioenergetic clocks pertain to the mitochondrial aspects of a cell. Both of these methodologies use a cell- or tissue-specific approach. While the accuracy of these estimations seem to vary by cell type, this does not disprove their validity. In fact, both approaches have elucidated or confirmed key aspects of aging—namely that various cells and tissues not only replicate but also age at different rates. And they do so, at least in part, due to exogenous or epigenetic factors. While these methodologies serve as valuable gauges of the health or functional status of a cell, both appear to be incomplete representations of biological aging of the person as a whole.

One of the most exciting discoveries in cellular rejuvenation, which was worthy of a 2012 Nobel Prize, came from Japanese stem-cell researcher Shinya Yamanaka. He and his research team identified four transcription factors (cellular proteins that regulate gene expression) that are capable of reprogramming mature adult cells and turning back their epigenetic clock to a younger embryonic state. Known commonly as Yamanaka Factors, these four genes have been successfully used to reprogram cells in mice, resulting in a significant extension in lifespan of these mice. Yamanaka's work has revolutionized stem cell therapy, leading to new stem cell treatments and techniques that are able to greatly increase our regenerative potential.

Despite these groundbreaking discoveries in stem cell science and cellular aging, we still don't have a set of biomarkers that gauges a person's overall biological age any better than their actual age. But the goal still remains. If we can find evidence of a biomarker or cluster of markers that accurately reflects biological aging, perhaps we can influence the master controls and turn back the clock on aging—or even prevent death.

Genetic Determinism and Epigenetics in Aging

Since the Human Genome Project was completed in 2003, there is still much uncertainty and debate among researchers about how the human genome carries out such an amazing array of complex function given that we have about half the number of protein-coding genes as a rice plant. And it now appears that perhaps more than 98 percent of our genome, known as "junk DNA," doesn't even code for proteins. Instead the junk DNA function as regulatory genetic switches, produce noncoding RNAs, and hold the chromosomes together.

In the last half of the 20th century, genetic determinism was the dominating paradigm. The idea was that the genes you inherit are the primary determining factor that guide your state of health, your odds of getting a specific disease, and your longevity. But in the past two decades, the prevailing paradigm has radically shifted to embrace the concept of epigenetics.

The prefix, *epi*, meaning "above," describes function that occurs above the level of the genes. This term characterizes changes not necessarily to the DNA or RNA codes themselves, but rather to the expression of the DNA or RNA. In other words, given a certain influence, an individual gene may increase or decrease expression based on the environmental signals. The most obvious empirical example of epigenetics can be seen from the observation of genetically identical twins. Over time, as each twin operates in different environments and engages in different thoughts, emotions, and behaviors, they eventually begin to look different or even sound different.

The story doesn't stop there, however. Despite our understanding of genetics and epigenetics, we cannot make the mistake and assume that all expression and function is guided solely by our genes. Recent research suggests that cells with their nucleus removed can survive for months and carry out complex functions despite not having the human genome present to direct cell function. There have been so many major illuminations in the past few decades that it is impossible to capture the totality of discovery. And still, despite all that has been uncovered by modern science, there is perhaps more confusion now than ever before when it comes to the biology of aging. Turns out, the closer we look, the more complexity we find.

THEORIES OF AGING

Currently, there are essentially two dominant categories of aging theories floating about Western science: programmed theories and damage theories. Some of these theories attempt to explain the biological mechanisms—how we age. Others instead opt for more of an evolutionary, philosophical, or teleological explanation of aging—why we age.

Programmed Theories

The general concept of the many programmed theories involves a biological clock that sets a limit on biological processes before death. Programmed theories seem to fit well with most ideas in evolutionary biology. After all, there is a predictable average and maximal lifespan within a given species. For example, humans live to about 80 years on average with a maximal lifespan of around 120 years by all available evidence. African elephants live to about 70 years old. Lions in the wild live to be about 20 years on average, while lions in captivity can live as long as 30 years. The lifespan of an individual can vary considerably given environmental conditions and lifestyle factors, but extreme outliers don't seem to exist. We don't see lions living to 80 years old, for example.

The most famous of the programmed theories is known as the Hayflick limit. Named in 1961 after Professor Leonard Hayflick, he demonstrated that a standard fetal cell will divide roughly 50 times in a laboratory cell culture before entering the cell death process known as apoptosis. Many researchers and scientists have even used the Hayflick limit postulate to calculate the maximum potential for human lifespan at 115 to 120 years. However, due to plenty of worthy criticism in recent years, explanation for the Hayflick limit is now thought to be a residual effect of telomere damage. (Recall that telomeres are small bits of genetic code that reside at the end of chromosomes that protect them from damage and provide greater stability to the DNA.) If the Hayflick limit is a residual effect of telomere damage, then it would fall into the category of damage theories, not programmed theories.

Another notable programmed theory of aging is antagonist pleiotropy. The central idea of this theory is that the same sets of genes responsible for sexual development and fertility are inextricably linked to the process of aging. Viewed through the lens of evolutionary biology, this means that sexual development and fertility provide a disadvantage to the *individual* (a shorter lifespan) but confers an evolutionary advantage to the *species* due to increased likelihood of reproduction. Evidence continues to mount for the antagonist pleiotropy theory, and it has attracted an increasing amount research in the last two decades. However, researchers still have yet to confirm the existence of a set of genes that can be solely identified as the master clock responsible for the aging program.

Damage Theories

The overall concept of the various damage theories center around internal processes that initiate damage and a build-up of cellular waste as part of normal, natural, living function. This leads to a cascade of damage to cellular architecture, genetic mutation, and reduction in overall healthy cell function. And the cumulative destruction over time prevents full repair and regeneration, resulting in senescence and ultimately cell death. Senescence is a marked shift in cell function toward reduction of cell division and increased cellular inflammation. So really, we have damage upon damage upon damage that impacts a variety of cellular components, cellular systems, and healthy genetic expression. And when too much damage is done, the cell is incapable of recovering and dies. Mitochondria, the tiny organelles inside our cells, tend to become central figures in most of the damage theories that exist today.

The variety of popular damage theories all stand on fairly solid scientific ground and do a great job of explaining the mechanisms of aging. All in all, each theory tends to carry some weight. But analyzed independently, they all seem to come up short. The primary limitation is that they fail to address the root mechanism or reason why all living beings must necessarily experience an inescapable decline of regeneration and loss of function. If the capacity for repair and regeneration exists in the genome, what prevents it from keeping up with damage? How do we have such an incredible capacity to build new tissue, repair damage, create complexity, and organize structure as we grow from zygote to embryo to child—and then that capability just starts losing steam, perhaps around puberty, to the point where the body can no longer keep up with damage that accumulates?

Fundamentally, the damage theories, while very helpful in describing various aging mechanisms—the *how*—have yet to provide sufficient evidence and explanation for the most important aging questions—the *why* or the *where*. It forces us back to the programmed theories in search of an unknown biological clock still hidden somewhere in the human body. The biological clock seems most plausible, but science can't seem to nail down where the master control is.

THE HOLOBIONT AND BEYOND

Contrary to the way mainstream science studies aging, it is helpful to take a step back and recognize the variety of players in this game of human life. Your body is a holobiont—a "superorganism"—an immense walking, talking rainforest of genetic material that coordinates, communicates, and responds to every perceived energetic stimulus it encounters. It is impossible to learn about disease or aging by studying a single component of the human body without factoring in the influence of the whole.

Within the microbiota, mitochondria, and human genetics, we have three distinct sets of genomes in the human body that are all working together to carry out function, maintain balance, and repair damaged parts. All these genomes are actually communicating with one another, constantly sending messages to one another to determine which genes the others should express to maintain homeostasis given the energetic environment they perceive.

What we're dealing with here is interspecies communication. Bacteria are talking to organelles and humans, and humans are talking to bacteria and organelles on a subcellular level. The language is energetic and quite complex, but researchers have identified many biochemical signals they use to accomplish this communication. For example, some gut microbes will produce things such as sulfide, hydrogen sulfide, secondary bile acids, nitric oxide, butyrate, or propionate that act as direct signals to influence mitochondrial function and DNA expression in the colon cells. Likewise, the mitochondria from colon cells will release reactive oxygen species (ROS), heat, and light that will send a cascading influence of factors that, in turn, modulate microbe function in the gut.

Researchers are still attempting to identify the countless metabolites and signals produced by microbes to get a better understanding of how they influence mitochondrial activity and human epigenetic expression. Because these bi-directional signals are so dynamic and influenced by just about every stimulus you can think of—exercise, diet, sleep, emotions, temperature, light, sound, microbes in the environment—it makes it very difficult to get a clear and total picture of what is really going on.

The key to understanding aging is that it's not just about the telomeres, it's not just the genes, it's not just the mitochondria or the microbiota or the cell membranes . . . It's all these things and more, collectively losing coherent function and accumulating damage over time. And because these signals determine the level of damage and repair going on in the body, we cannot discount the immense activity in search of a single, hypothetical golden key of aging. The contributors to a decline in biological function and increased aging are many.

The only real solution to improving health as you age is to take a truly integrated and holistic approach.

Chapter 2

EVERYTHING IS ENERGY, EVERYTHING IS CONNECTED

The day science begins to study nonphysical phenomena,
it will make more progress in one decade than in
all the previous centuries of its existence.

— Nikola Tesla

ENERGY AND EPIGENETICS

Your health is not controlled by your genes. Your health is an expression of everything you do, feel, think, believe, and interact with. There is an immense dynamic interaction between the microbiota, mitochondria, and your human DNA. It is the complex coordination of the genetic codes expressed by these three systems that is responsible for the totality of mechanistic biological function carried out in the body.

But genes cannot simply turn on and off by themselves. They have no ability to spontaneously self-express without a stimulus. No signal, no genetic function. The science of epigenetics explores the energetic conditions that regulate gene expression.

In essence, the genes and proteins that make up your micro-biota, mitochondria, and human cells are always perceiving and responding to energetic signals, be they consciously recognized or not. Your health or disease state, along with your rate of aging, is determined by the totality of the perceived internal and external energetic stimuli over time.

Not only do we see genes modulating expression when exposed to a changing environment, but as genes become exposed to novel environments and new stimuli, they also have the ability to mutate and adapt over time. In other words, you can funda-mentally change certain aspects of your DNA in order to better harmonize with a new environment. You actually have specific genes dedicated to recoding your own genome. And this gives you at least some ability to genetically adapt to your perceived environment.

Over many generations, adaptive genetic changes will occur, producing such physical effects. This genetically adaptive capa-bility is not only expressed in physical appearance, but also with respect to many systems at the cellular level. And let's not forget that mitochondria and microbiota also have some ability to adapt their genes to new environments as well.

This holobiont and epigenetic aspect of human biology is what allows you to be supremely adaptable to all perceived ener-getic signals in the environment, both in the short term and over the course of many generations. And while it is important not to discount your ability to adapt to an environment, there are limits to this adaptive capacity. For example, someone with red hair, light skin, and freckles will have a very limited capacity to adapt to the levels of solar radiation found at the equator. Excess exposure to solar radiation will lead to significant DNA damage in the skin, resulting in sunburn and potentially cancer. While this is an obvious example, it demonstrates that there are optimal and suboptimal diet and lifestyle choices you can make based on your unique constitution or genetic heritage.

HOLISTIC APPROACHES BEYOND NEWTONIAN BIOLOGY

When we look back at the popular aging theories, each appears to be a valuable piece of the same incomplete puzzle. They all begin with a strictly Newtonian-mechanics–based, materialistic premise in which the body acts like a complex machine that is intrinsically predestined to wear down as it carries out countless cellular tasks throughout life. But when we narrowly focus on any compartmentalized system or process in the body, we can lose sight of the fact that everything is operating concurrently, that the body systems are all connected, and many mechanisms of regulation and damage simultaneously exist.

Isn't it possible that all the programmed and damage theories of aging have some validity? It seems clear that they all hold essential biological aging truths. When combined, the theories certainly form a more complete and synergistic picture of the aging process than any of the theories on their own. And yet, collectively, they appear to still fall short of encapsulating the fundamental origins of biological aging.

For many practical reasons, scientific research tends to focus in on isolated aspects of function. But in so doing, it neglects the intelligent complexity of the body and the interrelated findings within other scientific fields of study. If we're able to move beyond siloed thinking, we have the opportunity to transcend and include the old concepts and frameworks. This opens up completely new paradigms of theory and possibility, allowing for a more holistic explanation to biology's big questions.

Scientific ideas can often look like the parable of the blind men and the elephant. A group of blind men come across an elephant for the first time, without knowing anything about this animal. The first man runs his hands across the body and says, "An elephant is like a large, rough wall." The second blind man grabs a tusk and exclaims, "Wrong, an elephant is like a smooth spear!" The third man runs his hands along the trunk and says, "No, an elephant is certainly rough, but it is more like a large hose." And yet the fourth man grabs an ear and says, "I agree, an elephant is very rough, but it is more like some kind of a fan." The larger picture is that all their realities are correct. *And* when all their experiences are put together, a new reality emerges. A more complete reality, revealing a greater truth.

This is analogous to all the partially complete aging theories. All the answers hold weight. But there is a value in thinking more comprehensively, particularly in the biological sciences. In order to get to the core of the aging issue, we must move beyond the Newtonian-mechanics–based, materialistic view of human biology. Otherwise, we will continue to get lost in the infinite depths of compartmentalized, biological materialism.

The field of physics, particularly quantum physics, has seen an explosion in new discoveries and updated theories. The pieces are slowly coming together with new understandings of concepts such as quantum entanglement, black holes, electromagnetism, quantum tunneling, the electrical properties of water, and torsion fields. Along with these advances, the intersection of physics and biology has drawn significant interest by those who have been unsatisfied with the lack of answers provided by biochemistry alone.

Over the past few decades, Western scientific research has been dedicating more resources to the study of biophysics. We've now seen experiments that explore the biophysics of meditation, the energy storage capacity of water, how thoughts influence biochemistry, the influence of sound and light on genetic expression, and the study of consciousness itself. And while the existing paradigms are fighting to stay alive, it is through the lens of biophysics where we begin to see new realities emerge.

BIOLOGICAL COHERENCE

If we turn toward physics for a succinct definition of *coherence*, it can be described as the optimal state of energy efficiency and harmonious activity in a system. Biological coherence, then, can be described as the ability of a biological system to optimize harmonious activity and energy efficiency.

Because the body is composed of nested hierarchical structures, coherence can be exhibited across all space and time scales. From the quantum level to the cellular level and to the body as a whole, each can exhibit coherence within each level and with the whole. At all levels, improved biological coherence results in a more effective storage and transfer of energy and information in a system that results in improved communication, efficiency, order, and harmony. When coherence is reduced, we lose communication, efficiency, order, and harmony, which results in an increase of dysfunction, damage, and eventually death.

At the cellular level, coherence induces harmonious and efficient communication between the mitochondria, nuclear genome, intercellular milieu, and extracellular matrix. In this perfect, theoretical condition, energy transfer is optimized and the damage from oxidation is offset by appropriate signaling required to initiate life-affirming mechanisms such as cellular defense, apoptosis, autophagy, mitophagy, telomerase activity, stem cell activation, dedifferentiation, and redifferentiation. I say theoretically because perfect coherence is likely impossible. But by increasing coherent activity of the many biological processes, you foster greater repair, recycling, and regeneration on every level, which maximizes vitality as you age.

The unimaginably complex form and function of life is sustained through a constant supply of energy. It is the energetic fields and electric charges that animate sub-cellular proteins and enzymes to carry out specific functions in response to perceived environmental signals. Electric charge is responsible for protein folding, energy transfer, gene expression, and regeneration. And it is the cell membranes that play such an important role in creating a charge barrier, separating water inside the cell and the water outside the cell. This is one of the reasons cell membranes are often a focus of longevity research and theories of aging. There are thousands of proteins imbedded in cell membranes that serve a crucial role in transmitting energetic signals from the extracellular space to the thousands of cellular components that carry out form, function, and behavior of a cell at any given time.

Because human beings are open energetic systems that maintain a continuous exchange of energy and information with the environment, anything that influences electric charge will consequently influence movement and biological activity on the physical level. It is through this mechanism that we can begin to understand how unseen energies such as sound, light, magnetism, atmospheric pressure, thoughts, emotions, and beliefs can influence our biology. All have the intrinsic capacity to interact with energetic fields, influence electric charge, modulate gene expression, and even recode existing genes.

Just as classical physics has made room for the study of quantum physics, I invite you to recognize that your biology operates not only in a classical, material way but also in a nonmaterial, energetic way. There's a beautiful saying apocryphally attributed to Einstein: "We're slowed-down sound and light waves. A walking bundle of frequencies tuned into the cosmos."

Undoubtedly you've felt the effects of these unseen environmental energies on your biology. It can be quite palpable. Ever felt a loud base beat rattle your body at a concert? Maybe you've had to give a speech in front of an audience and all of a sudden, for no reason other than your own conditioned thoughts and subconscious beliefs, you start getting hot and flush. Your heart races and your palms get sweaty. In the *European Journal of Preventive Cardiology*, researchers observed a significant reduction in heart attacks in the three days following a new moon. And, in 2011, the National Institutes of Health (NIH) published a study demonstrating a highly significant increase in the severity of illness and aggressive behavior associated with phases of the moon. It is likely due to these observable changes in behavior that the term *lunatic* originated in the late 13th century. These are just a few examples of how unseen energies have an effect on our minds and bodies.

If you can open up fully to this level of reality, new possibilities emerge for you to explore how subtle energies induced by sound, light, magnetism, thoughts, beliefs, and emotions may be affecting your health or disease state.

INFORMATIONAL FIELDS

How is it that a human being comes into existence with such mindblowing complexity and function? How does the first liver cell come to be? And how does the organism know exactly when to develop and where to place the first liver cells? Research has identified the role of retroviruses in some of these mechanisms, to be sure, but what guides the process and timing of such coordinated development from a single-celled zygote to the presence of a highly complex and ordered being? How is it that nearly every child moves through the intricate stages of motor development in near-identical fashion and timing?

Instinct and development are described as genetically "hard-wired." While true to some degree, this description stops short of explaining how information becomes hard-wired across an entire species. Furthermore, being able to explain the physical mechanisms should not be mistaken for the fundamental source of the information.

Recall that genes require an animating force. This animating force is electrical charge at the physical level. But there also must be some sort of information or intelligence involved. Genetic material is incapable of coordinating complex form and function on its own. Heredity of form and information, it seems, is rooted in both genes and an informational field.

While the full biological picture remains fuzzy and incomplete, the latest scientific theories consistently point to a very real and non-material explanation for these biological enigmas. The biologist Rupert Sheldrake posits that organizing informational fields exist that help guide the development, form, and behavior across a given species. This "morphic field," as he calls it, has inherent memory of repeatable behaviors or habits that are consciously communicated through a resonant informational field that can be referenced by the entire species. While this theory is not broadly entertained, there is evidence that suggests Sheldrake may be on to something.

Other theories of informational fields include Carl Jung's idea of archetypes and the human collective unconscious. Quantum physics and biophysics are converging on the idea that the universe and all life is likely acted upon, produced by, and connected by a unifying, holographic, and self-referencing energetic field that is coherent and harmonic at all scales of existence. The work of world-renowned physicists Dr. Nikolai Kozyrev and Dr. Claude Swanson suggest that torsion fields are likely the interactive medium through which our thoughts, emotions, and awareness can "step outside" of time to instantaneously influence biology both locally and remotely.

Each framework seems to be pointing to very similar ideas. It appears as though it is the interaction of conscious and subconscious awareness with some kind of energetic or informational field through which all biological mind–matter interactions occur. Physicist Sir James Jeans wrote in 1931: "Today there is a wide measure of agreement, which on the physical side of science approaches almost to unanimity, that the stream of knowledge is heading towards a non-mechanical reality; the universe begins to look more like a great thought than like a great machine. Mind no longer appears as an accidental intruder into the realm of matter; we are beginning to suspect that we ought rather to hail it as a creator and governor of the realm of matter."

In the scientific realm alone, we have theories of morphic fields, the quantum field, the collective unconscious, and torsion fields. All these frameworks circle around the idea of an intelligent field that interacts with physical reality. But even a divine architect or intelligent field must have the correct circumstance to carry out her vision. In nature, healthy apples will grow only in an energetic environment that is harmonious for an apple. Humans are no different.

When coupled with the optimal energetic environment, your unique health code can be efficiently expressed. The information and pattern already exists, and you will express biological coherence when the energetic field of your inner and outer environment is in harmony with the informational field that guides your biology. In other words, health is the result of aligning with your unique constitution and nature as a whole.

A NEW LOOK AT AGING

Let's now go back to our attempt to define aging. With our understanding of the holobiont and biological coherence, I propose a new definition: aging is the real-time process of losing biological coherence on any level, resulting in an inability to adapt, repair, and regenerate to the degree necessary to overcome the accumulation of damage.

Per this definition, we can have a toggling of both aging and regeneration happening inside the same cell. Or we might have a fast rate of aging in the heart and a slower rate of aging in the liver, for example. It is the varying rates of aging in a cell, tissue, or system, accounted for in this definition, that allows for organ-specific conditions such as cardiac arrest, kidney failure, type 2 diabetes, cirrhosis, stroke, or Alzheimer's disease. There is nothing wrong with the genes, per se. Rather it is localized, loss of biological coherence that accounts for the organ-specific issue.

Depending on changing circumstances and environmental conditions, an aging cell or organ may subsequently improve its coherence in such a way that may foster repair, recycling, and regeneration and reduce damage. Because the entire body is connected, when one tissue or system is weak, the body systems will attempt to compensate in order to maintain homeostasis and function. And in so doing, it will lose systemic coherence as total energy efficiency decreases.

Additionally, our definition suggests that aging can be happening at any point in life—in youth and beyond. This helps solve the riddle of "when does aging begin?" To that we can say: as soon as regeneration and repair cannot keep up with damage. With this conceptual framework, we might approach aging beyond just a longevity-focused mind-set. We don't want to add more sub-optimal, "damaged" years to our lives; the goal is to maximize biological coherence to the degree we are able as we grow older.

The question is: Can we rebound and reverse the localized effects of aging or will it accumulate further? The more biological aging occurs in a cell or tissue, the harder it becomes to reverse, and thus, biological aging will tend to accelerate. In other words, damage in a given tissue leads to more damage in that tissue or the system as a whole.

In a way, we might view the body's biological processes and expression as analogous to a flawless manufacturing assembly line. You only need to concern yourself with general parameters and limitations of your assembly line and *what raw material you're feeding into it*. Then by tuning in, feeling, listening, and observing the quality of the final product, you can tweak and adjust your inputs.

There may be value in learning each of the assembly line's processes. But if you aren't aware of all the inputs and your entire system's parameters and limitations, being an expert on the processes won't get you very far. Instead, you're more likely to assign flaw to a flawless process. This is where most of traditional Western medical thinking resides. It looks for for major flaws in a system with near-perfect potential. It tends to mistake incoherence and imbalance for inherent defects.

Chapter 3

RESOLVING DISEASE OR BUILDING HEALTH

*It is no measure of health to be well
adjusted to a profoundly sick society.*

— JIDDU KRISHNAMURTI

In my private health practice over the past several years, I've seen many chronic conditions, including women in their 30s losing their hair, men in their 20s unable to get erections, and children as young as 3 with food intolerances and digestive issues. So many in the U.S. are dealing with food sensitivities, immune system dysregulation, digestive issues, sleep problems, and mental-emotional challenges. While cancer, heart disease, and neurodegenerative disorders capture most of the headlines and emotional draw, it is the growing cluster of low-grade, inflammatory conditions that should be cluing us in to the deteriorating health of the youth populations in many industrialized nations. Statistically speaking, chronic disease is increasing dramatically, affecting younger populations at alarming rates.

The United States is staring at an epidemic of chronic disease with the potential to bankrupt the nation and unravel a global economic recession. According to the Centers for Disease Control and Prevention, as much as 90 percent of the $4.1 trillion we spend annually on health care is allotted to treating chronic health conditions. We're told by a medical establishment that it's normal to spend our adult years in pain—be it physical, mental, or emotional. While these symptoms and conditions appear to be common, we need not accept them as normal.

There is no question that traditional Western medicine has saved countless lives in the form of acute care. But where the system doesn't fare so well is in the true resolution of chronic illness. Unfortunately, the cost of extending lives through the traditional medical model appears to be long-term symptom management, pharmaceutical dependency, side effects, and greater incidence and severity of chronic disease.

Due to this systemic limitation, an increasing number of individuals have been turning to physicians, practitioners, and coaches who offer more holistic and integrative methods of managing and resolving chronic disease. I was fortunate to find tremendous clinicians and mentors to guide my understanding as a practitioner, honing my ability to support clients when modern medicine failed. Through this process, I learned one of the greatest philosophical and practical lessons: there is a distinct difference between addressing disease and cultivating health.

No amount of disease resolution can actually create health. Using a house fire as a metaphor, it would be akin to believing you can repair the house by putting out the fire. Yet Western medicine focuses on diagnosing and treating disease, with almost no focus on teaching the principles of vitality and a healthy lifestyle, let alone where health originates in the first place. It appears that in our quest to reduce early death, we have forgotten the importance of health.

Technological progress grants us greater ability to perform medical miracles with our modern acute-care practices. If we can find a way to combine ancient wisdom with modern technology, lifespan and health span will rise in tandem like never before. But we must shift our approach, take back our individual power, and reclaim sovereignty over our health. True healing can only be realized when we give the body and mind an opportunity to thrive by creating the physical, mental, and emotional, and energetic environment to support the innate healing process.

SHIFTING THE PARADIGM OF HEALTH CARE

Technological advancements over the past 100 years in the West have undoubtedly been the largest contributor to the monumental increases in lifespan and average life expectancy. Unparalleled prosperity pulled people out of poverty like never before. Greater financial independence allowed individuals to live on their own, away from family. Personal gardens and farmers markets were no longer required as supermarkets became the norm. Vigorous movement and nonstop physical labor was no longer a necessary part of daily life—a stark contrast to those born just two or three generations prior. Herbal concoctions and home remedies were swapped for the latest and greatest pharmaceutical drug to hit the market.

We've gotten so caught up in the promise of technological innovation, we forgot to ask ourselves in what direction we desire to go and why. On the whole, we've become blind to the fact that just because we could, doesn't mean we should. Without a guiding philosophy or big-picture teleology, we continue to run the risk of creating new, unforeseen health challenges with each existing problem we aim to solve. Perhaps the dominating philosophy of the traditional Western medical system requires a complete overhaul to address the core issues we currently face.

Fundamentally, we have lost confidence in the innate wisdom of our own body and mind to do the healing. We have become blind to the signals the body, mind, and emotions are constantly sending that indicate something is out of alignment. There is immense and invaluable information encoded in the pain, inflammation, depression, dry skin, high blood pressure, fatigue, and the many other symptoms one can experience. We learned to rely on doctors, machines, drugs, news media, supplements—anything other than ourselves. After all, it's easy to buy into the idea that we're not in control of our health.

There is a real opportunity now to regain your ability to decipher the codes your body sends. However, if you ignore your biological "check engine lights," full breakdown is just a matter of time. The immense wisdom of your body will keep sending these signals and knocking louder until you either address the underlying issues or disaster forces your hand. The choice is yours.

We've been conditioned to focus on the disease with which we've been labeled. As a result, it becomes easy to lose sight of the fact that we have the power to heal on our own. With a little practice, you can learn how to listen to the subtle cues the body and mind are sending. Doing so will cultivate a profound level of awareness, giving you the ability to navigate the constantly changing environmental and lifestyle conditions, moment by moment, for the rest of your life.

If you want a greater health span and lifespan, the first step is to make the decision to create a new reality for yourself. Your beliefs and intentions are powerful. With the humility to accept responsibility for your current situation and the courage to change it, you unlock radical new possibility.

AN INTEGRATIVE PERSPECTIVE—MOVING BEYOND THE ACUTE-CARE MODEL

The prevailing Western paradigm views the various parts of the body as distinct and separate. It identifies the piece that appears to be causing an issue, assigns a disease label to the cluster of symptoms, then attempts to address the symptoms with medication, psychiatric treatments, supplements, and/or surgeries. This can be a very effective way to halt the progression of acute symptoms, which is how the methodology primarily evolved—to deal with things like battle wound complications, soft tissue damage, organ failures, and other physical traumas. But this acute-care model of disease management is insufficient and increasingly ineffective at addressing the chronic physical, mental, and emotional conditions plaguing the industrialized world.

When an acute care model is used to address every minor ailment or illness that arises, we rob our body of the opportunity to build up natural immunity and greater resiliency. Ultimately, this myopic focus on diagnosing disease and managing symptoms has created a pill for every ill. These outdated methods are turning away thousands of disappointed and disillusioned doctors in search of a new method of practice that allows them to actually help people overcome their chronic conditions.

As patients, we have been trained to accept this failing mode of operation. Seeing the doctor has become like taking your car to the mechanic. You go in to inspect the part of your body that's "malfunctioning," thinking that's where the problem lies. But the fundamental issue cannot be resolved by addressing only the individual parts without consideration of the whole, including the entire body, mind, emotions, energy, health history, environment, lifestyle, and even family history.

Innovative medical approaches—complementary, integrative, and functional medicine—work holistically to resolve disease and provide solutions for underlying conditions. However, in the process of evaluation, there can still be a tendency to diagnose a group of symptoms so you can give it a specific disease label. This makes it easier to quantify biological functions and qualify the biological responses and accompanying symptoms. However, it may create an intellectual obstacle for the practitioner with respect to where the real problems lie. In addition, any objective identification or label can create a placebo or psychosomatic obstacle for the patient, because it reinforces the idea that the fundamental issue is an error of the physical body—that there is something "wrong" with the patient.

What's more, if an attempted fix does not help restore balance in a way that is coherent or harmonious with our entire biological system, then it may exacerbate the existing core issues by adding more imbalances to the mix. There is a lot to consider. But failure to thoroughly investigate all aspects of health, with the intent of restoring balance and harmony to the system, is why I believe so many people struggle to find solutions to their chronic conditions, let alone thrive into old age.

ADDRESSING THE TERRAIN, NOT JUST THE ROOTS

While there are undoubtedly instances of known major genetic disorders, the *origin* of most chronic illness is not a malfunctioning tissue, organ, or gene. In many cases, the core pattern of chronic illness can be found to originate in the conscious and subconscious mind along with how we're thinking, feeling, and interacting with our environment. These core patterns can prime the physical body toward disharmony that shows up as imbalanced immune function, poor detoxification pathways, chaotic autonomic nervous system function, poor digestive function, hypothyroidism, low nutrient absorption, leaky barriers, excess inflammation, etc. Imbalanced and disharmonious function in the body can then create greater susceptibility to infections, gut microbiota imbalances, mitochondrial disorders, poor epigenetic expression, and any other "disease" marker that can be tested, identified, and traced.

Aside from true genetic abnormalities, chronic conditions are always downstream effects of *how* we are living in and perceiving the world. While dysfunctions may be present in the body, their origins are rarely due to the inability of our bodies to properly operate. In order to heal, we must focus on the internal and external environment, not the syndromes and symptoms.

There is a lot of talk these days about getting to the root cause of disease. While I appreciate the metaphor, it could use some tweaking. If a tree is sick, the sole solution isn't to nurture healthy roots. We must look to the soil ecosystem and assess whether the above-ground environment is suitable for the tree to thrive. To cultivate health in the entirety of the tree, it is important to address the entire terrain while *also* nurturing the roots.

When it comes to chronic illness, there are three superficial levels of symptoms before you get to the "terrain," using our analogy above. It can be effective to nurture, balance, and influence factors on Levels 1 through 3. But until you address Levels 4 through 6, there will be symptoms up the ladder.

THE HIERARCHY OF SYMPTOMS

- **Level 1** [the labels]: hypertension, diabetes, rheumatoid arthritis, Hashimoto's thyroiditis, kidney disease, eczema, etc.

- **Level 2** [the markers]: high blood pressure, high hemoglobin A1C, elevated inflammatory markers, low thyroid hormone, low GFR, etc.

- **Level 3** [the expressions]: mitochondrial damage, gastrointestinal inflammation, poor cellular communication, chronic inflammation, anxiety, depression, structural misalignment, etc.

- **Level 4** [the behaviors]: improper diet and exercise, poor sleep, smoking, shallow breathing, social isolation, overworking, self-harm, etc.

- **Level 5** [the thoughts, feelings, beliefs]: anger, fear, guilt, shame, apathy, disappointment, ignorance, low self-worth, insecurity, etc.

- **Level 6** [the core wounds]: traumatic birth, developmental ruptures, significant emotional trauma, physical trauma, inherited traumas, disharmonious environment, etc.

When you understand this framework, you'll be far less likely to get stuck at the superficial levels in which the traditional Western medical system operates. With greater familiarity of the deeper levels of healing, you'll likely find that interaction with your inner and outer environment in the form of thoughts, feelings, beliefs, and behavior is where you have immense power to create impactful change to your health and well-being.

Modern medicine seeks to address the high-level disease label the patient is given—the type 2 diabetes, heartburn, migraines, dermatitis, and the like. Sometimes medication is prescribed directly in response to surface-level symptoms. Otherwise, basic lab testing may be suggested.

If we look deeper to Level 2, we can often find imbalanced biological markers that reside in the body and are associated with the surface-level symptoms and diagnoses. These biological imbalances that might show up on lab tests include things such as elevated blood pressure, low testosterone, high blood sugar levels, elevated liver enzymes, and low thyroid hormone.

As we continue to go deeper to Level 3, it becomes possible to identify the fundamental biological symptoms of imbalanced expression at the level of mitochondrial function, microbial ecosystem, cellular communication, and maladaptive epigenetic expression. We now have metabolomics testing, gut microbiota testing, intercellular testing, and the testing of specific epigenetic markers. This level of testing can detect markers associated with imbalanced biological expression of the body and sometimes offer enough information to guide you toward strategies for restoring optimal function. But oftentimes, this level of testing falls short because it still fails to answer: "Why?" In order to answer this most fundamental question, we have to look to Level 4 and beyond.

Levels 4 and 5 are the domain of thinking, feeling, beliefs, and behavior. To realize optimal health and harmony, it is imperative to identify behaviors that are likely contributing to suboptimal epigenetic expression and imbalanced markers on lab tests— behaviors such as improper diet, poor sleep, chemical exposure, excessive alcohol, social isolation, lack of exercise, or perhaps too much exercise, among others.

What further complicates the issue with these behavioral patterns is the origin of the behavior. Unhealthy behavior may be a direct result of a core wound, or it may be due to ignorance, or how you think or feel, or even what your conditioned beliefs are. Behavior is much more complicated than most of us recognize. Oftentimes it can be so hard to imagine why somebody else would continuously behave in a way that is clearly causing harm. But behavior is rarely guided by logic. In fact, the fascinating field of behavioral economics demonstrates how predictably irrational we all are in the face of seemingly straightforward economic choices. As it turns out, our behavior is heavily influenced by our subconscious thoughts, conditioned beliefs, and patterned emotions. Oftentimes, behavior, even unhealthy behavior, is guided by the attempt to get a fundamental need met. Thanks in large part to researchers such as Bruce Lipton, Bessel van der Kolk, Joe Dispenza, Gabor Maté, and many others, we are now starting to understand just how thoughts and emotions translate to behavior, cellular function, and epigenetic expression.

Finally, we get to Level 6, the core wounds that set the stage for most illness and disease. Inevitably, core wounds have to do with an overwhelming experience or recurring conditions that have triggered an acute, adaptive survival response in the body and mind. When this adaptive response is chronically expressed, even in the absence of threat, it will usually lead to maladaptive patterns and disharmony in the body and mind. It's important to note here that your mind and body aren't faulty; they are simply caught in a pattern of operation, one that was necessary to cope with a previous (or perhaps ongoing) experience that exceeds your capacity to fully process it. With a keen awareness, one can always find various forms of conditioning, developmental rupture, trauma, lack of secure emotional attachment, or an overall disharmonious environment at some point in life—often at multiple points throughout life. Eliminating the overwhelming experience or trigger that created the adaptive survival pattern is generally beneficial. But the truth is, even when the triggers are no longer present, our body and mind can get pattern-locked as they continue to run the old adaptive patterns in the form of thoughts, emotions, beliefs, and behaviors. And these patterns tend to impair function if they are no longer required in the context of a new environment or if there is a more optimal way of being that can be expressed. (We'll dive into this topic a little deeper in later chapters.)

As you can see, the symptom hierarchy has many levels beyond 1 through 3 that are usually attended to. Many times, you may find solutions on a superficial level and get stuck, thinking that's where the story ends. Usually, there are deeper aspects to uncover and more work to be done to restore biological coherence. One of the greatest traps you can get pulled into is successfully finding a supplement, protocol, herb, therapy, or drug that can suppress or even remedy your symptoms while never getting to the deeper etiology of what led to or is causing the imbalance. Without understanding the real cause and what might need to change, it is not uncommon for imbalance and overt symptoms to return. If, however, you are able to truly understand the reasons your symptoms arose, bringing the body back into balance with natural means is much more likely to result in lasting health.

Remedies to chronic health issues at Level 1 usually involve pharmaceutical drugs and surgeries. Remedies at Levels 2 and 3 often include a change in diet, supplements, and herbs. Remedies at Levels 4 and 5 involve recognizing and working to change the conscious and subconscious thoughts, emotions, and behaviors that are contributing to your symptoms. Finally, the most illusive and intensive work lives at Level 6, which involves processing and integrating the many overwhelming experiences we've been unable to handle. Processing these experiences allows us to transform misperceptions and let go of the health-impairing mental and biological patterns that limit our ability to be optimally healthy. Through this deep inner work, we have the opportunity to become more aligned, embodied, and truly empowered. This book will help you navigate the entire symptom hierarchy so you can discover how to optimize your health, increase well-being, and thrive as you age.

A NEW PHILOSOPHY OF HEALING

Throughout life, we will all be faced with circumstances that we don't particularly enjoy. We'll continue to have many points of frustration, fear, anger, disease, depression, anxiety, and pain. Whenever these undesirable conditions and states arise, we have two options: accept our victimhood, or choose a more conscious participation and ownership of the situation.

In every instance of discomfort, we have an opportunity to transform the chaos into coherence; disharmony into harmony; pain into love. We are alchemists at our core. To quote Carl Jung, "There is no birth of consciousness without pain." Pain itself is the manifestation of consciousness awakening to the pattern of disharmony. As such, pain is the beginning of the healing process, and our symptoms are divine messengers sent by the body and mind to help wake us up.

Pain is just healing in disguise. If you are humble enough to listen to the feeling and courageous enough to walk the path, pain can be a brilliant teacher and one of the greatest gifts you'll ever receive. I realize it may sound callous or absurd to someone with, for example, rheumatoid arthritis or Crohn's disease that pain can be a great gift. But as you speak to individuals who experience total healing and remission of their conditions, you very often find there is a common recognition that the pain was indeed a gift that led them to a beautiful new life path and recognition of a more aligned and integrated truth. On the other side of healing, there is a stark realization that the suffering was rough but worth it. But while in the midst of the struggle, it can be challenging to see the light at the end of the tunnel.

For most of us, there exists a strong desire to push the pain away, proclaiming, "It is not mine. I do not want it." But if we are brave enough to accept responsibility for our current state of being, no matter how it might have come to be or who might have wronged us, we instantly create a subconscious shift that becomes an empowered invitation for massive transformation. The beautiful truth is that each of us already has everything we need to get beyond our pain and suffering.

However, if we are drugging, numbing, or ignoring pain in any way, we are merely shooting the messenger and turning our back on the opportunity for consciousness to awaken to a disharmonious pattern. Whether the coping strategy is of natural or synthetic means, we lose the conscious feedback loop. Of course, there are times when pain or disability is so pervasive and hindering that management is an important piece of the larger objective. But if the management is at the expense of bringing awareness to the true imbalance, over time the feedback loop will become more intense and perhaps present itself in a novel way. In other words, the pain and the symptoms progress or manifest in new places if the maladaptive patterns are not addressed.

Oftentimes, to truly heal, you must put yourself first, just as a flight attendant instructs you to put your oxygen mask on before you assist others in an in-flight emergency. The residual effect of transforming your health ripples through your family, community, and social network with a magnitude that is impossible to truly grasp. When you improve your mental, emotional, and physical well-being, you implicitly give permission and inspire others around you to do the same. It is the least selfish thing you can do because you cultivate greater capacity to lend your time, energy, and resource to others, especially those who depend on you or look to you for guidance. Your healing is one of the greatest gifts you can give the world because more of YOU can emerge to express your unique genius by living your dream.

WHAT IS YOUR INTENTION?

It is a commonly held belief that if my body and mind are working well enough and I feel okay now, I can go on doing exactly what I'm doing without having to worry about changing anything. Most of us learn this lesson the hard way as we eventually wake up to a crisis and only then do we start becoming conscious of what might be out of alignment. In fact, it took me 30 years and a lot of suffering to figure this out. And I still have yet to fully embody this realization. Many of us take better care of our cars than we do our bodies—scheduling regular checkups, getting the oil changed on time, replacing brake pads, rotating the tires, and the like. It seems rather foolish to put off your oil change until the engine seizes up. And yet, that's the approach many of us take with our health and well-being.

One of the ways to minimize the pain and suffering that can come from this conditioned way of being is to get clear on your primary dream or intention for your life in this moment. If you don't have a reason to evolve that is greater than the problem you are trying to solve, you're much less likely to achieve your objective. As psychologist Jerry Wesch said so well, "If you have a big enough dream, you don't need a crisis." By defining a clear intention or dream, you not only identify a North star to which you can orient your life, but you also create an attractive force—something pulling you in a direction that holds great meaning and creates happiness.

Start by creating a roadmap of your dream life. Where do you want to go and who do you want to be? The process of setting an intention begins to organize your conscious thoughts, beliefs, ideas, behaviors, and awareness to give you a better sense of where you are now and the vision of what you want to create as you consciously give your whole self passionately into freewill. One of the keys to identifying your dream is to find something that holds tremendous meaning for you—something that gives you profound joy and elicits a sense of gratitude. Friedrich Nietzsche famously said, "He whose life has a why can bear almost any how." In the context of your purpose or dream, this *why* that Nietzsche refers to might be thought of as your soul's dream or heart's desire.

Even if you don't know your precise life mission, by starting to plot the path and adjusting along the way, you'll find greater meaning in this human existence. Your dream or objective should also feel real, tangible, and achievable. Once you are clear on your dream, connect with it often and keep it front and center in your awareness. You might notice over time, it starts to lose meaning or shift in its importance. In this case, you can reevaluate and connect with a new dream or objective if it feels aligned.

There is tremendous self-healing potential that exists within you. The remainder of this book will provide a framework of health principles that, when implemented, have the power to unlock the body's timeless wisdom so you can express your unique health code and increase your well-being.

PART II

MOVING BEYOND LONGEVITY: INCREASING YOUR HEALTH SPAN

Chapter 4

SLEEP, LIGHT, AND CIRCADIAN RHYTHM

*A human body can think thoughts, play a piano, kill germs,
remove toxins, make a baby all at once. Once it's doing that,
your biological rhythms are actually mirroring the symphony
of the universe because you have circadian rhythms, seasonal
rhythms, tidal rhythms; you know, they mirror everything
that is happening in the whole universe.*

— MICHIO KAKU, ASTROPHYSICIST

It is hard to overstate the value of sleep and its role in maintaining health, recovering from illness, and extending life. The issues created by chronic poor sleep are too many to list in total—from weight gain to poor insulin regulation, increased inflammation, heart conditions, poor cognition, thyroid problems, a disrupted microbiome, adrenal dysregulation, hormonal imbalances, infertility, the list is endless. Tatsuo Kakinohana of Okinawa, at the age of 82, told me, "Even when we got sick, we rarely went to see a doctor. We healed by sleeping." This wisdom was echoed by 83-year-old Ayako Toguchi when she said, "The most important thing is balance in your way of eating, sleeping, and work. If there is imbalance, you will get sick." Research consistently shows that if you don't get optimal sleep, everything just breaks down faster.

Most repair and regeneration of the body and brain occurs during sleep. Sleep is when the cerebral spinal fluid clears metabolic waste out of the brain through the glymphatic system, a deeply important process to protect against dementia and Alzheimer's, for example. The brain also improves its communication and creates new muscle memory. Sleep enhances immune system function and improves balance. Short-term memory shifts to long-term, and the brain makes new neural connections. Hormone function is optimized and balanced due to proper hypothalamic-pituitary function. When you get proper sleep, the entire body is in cleaning, repair, and regeneration mode.

THE SLEEP CYCLES

There are two primary modes that make up a sleep cycle: non-rapid eye movement (non-REM) followed by rapid eye movement (REM). While there is variation in sleep architecture based on living conditions and climates, a night of good sleep in modern society tends to consist of four or five distinct cycles of approximately 90 minutes each.

Each non-REM cycle has four stages. Stage 1 is the lightest sleep. Stages 3 and 4 are the deepest, during which most of the body's restoration, recovery, and growth occurs.

For the typical young adult, REM sleep tends to account for about 20 percent of total sleep time. The REM phase is associated with memory consolidation, learning, creativity, and dreaming. Neurotransmitters that determine your mood the next day also get replenished and balanced in a big way during REM sleep.

HOW MUCH SLEEP DO YOU NEED?

Research has demonstrated time and again that the lack of sleep predicts all-cause mortality. In other words, the shorter your sleep, the shorter your life—statistically speaking. Studies show that just one night of poor sleep results in a dramatic reduction of natural killer cells, a critical aspect of immune function that keeps cancer in check, among other things.

When I asked the elders if they had any sleep troubles now or in their younger years, there just wasn't much to say. Not a single elder I spoke with around the world had any sleep troubles. It just wasn't an issue for them or people they knew. This is in stark contrast to industrialized nations. According to recent surveys, the average American adult only gets about 6.5 hours of sleep each night. In the early 1940s, it is estimated that Americans were getting around 7.9 hours of sleep per night on average.

Our sleeping needs change throughout life. Infants, children, teenagers, young adults, and elderly adults all have completely different sleep patterns, as you've probably noticed. While the typical adult will generally require seven to nine hours of sleep, some people require a little less, while others tend to need a little more. But the amount of sleep you actually need each night is completely dependent on what your body is craving. If you're sleep deprived, sick, pregnant, or have had a physically active day, your body might just crave more sleep in order to rejuvenate appropriately.

Research is pretty clear, however, that consistently getting less than seven hours of sleep has deleterious effects. Everything breaks down when we start to experience sleep issues, and eventually it starts to affect your daily life. You can't think as well, and memory suffers. You're more likely to get sick. Your ability to regulate blood sugar is disrupted and hunger hormones go awry, causing you to make poor eating choices. Your mood might shift as neurotransmitter balance is lost, creating a higher propensity to experience depression and anxiety. You're quicker to anger and tip into emotional stress as the activity of your prefrontal cortex is reduced and the emotional centers of the brain are more activated. All your emotional states can be completely altered with poor sleep. Your likelihood of physical injury increases, and recovery from all chronic diseases is undoubtedly hampered.

Studies have shown that, as a result of daylight savings time, when we turn our clocks back in the spring and most people lose an hour of sleep, we see a 24 percent increase in the number of heart attacks. In the fall, when most people tend to gain an hour of sleep, there is a 21 percent decrease in the number of heart attacks. There is no cell, tissue, or organ that is not affected by poor sleep, be it chronic or acute.

DETERMINING YOUR OWN SLEEP NEEDS

The elders we met in Ikaria, Sardinia, Okinawa, and Costa Rica were raised in an environment that required little thought when it came to sleep hygiene and nightly routine. They had few barriers between them and an excellent night's sleep. When I asked 35-year-old Javier Armijo if he knew whether any of his older Costa Rican relatives had any sleep issues he said, "Let me think about it, man . . . I don't think so. Well, the only guy I know who has a little bit of a problem sleeping right now is me because I have a new business that is taking a lot from me." *How American of him*, I thought.

Many of those who struggle with sleep are now turning to modern technology. High-tech consumer products on the market help individuals track not only sleep time but also sleep quality. Many of these wearable devices and apps compile multiple data points—including heart rate variability, pulse, temperature, and movement—to assess your sleep patterns. This can be a useful method to start understanding how your mood and behavior throughout the day is affecting your sleep.

There is an additional method that does not require the use of technology, however. With the practice of bringing mindful awareness to how you feel in the morning and throughout the day, you will be able to gauge your sleep and better recognize the subtle shifts of your internal state and how the external environment might be affecting you. Ask yourself the following:

- When you wake up, take notice of how well rested you feel. Are you able to jump out of bed or do you feel sluggish?

- Do you have energy throughout the day or is your body begging for a nap?

- How is your mood, decision making, and emotional state?

- Do you start feeling tired and ready for bed between 8 and 10 P.M. or are you still wide awake?

Regardless of whether you use sleep tracking technology to aid you, this level of awareness will better inform you about how your lifestyle is impacting your sleep and vice versa.

UNDERSTANDING BIOLOGICAL RHYTHMS

In 2017, the Nobel Prize in Physiology or Medicine was awarded to three Americans for their discoveries of the molecular mechanisms that control circadian rhythms. The word *circadian* comes from the Latin word *circa,* meaning "around," and *dias,* meaning "day." Since life began to form on this planet, every organism has had to adapt to the effects produced by the rotation, orbit, and axial tilt of Earth and the movement of other celestial bodies. This ability to predict and alter function based on the daily and seasonal fluctuations in light and temperature is crucial for all life.

We now know that every cell, tissue, and organ in your body is being guided by the 24-hour cycle of day and night, like a ticking clock. Practitioners of Ayurveda and Chinese medicine have been following this philosophy for thousands of years. And it's wonderful to see modern science now showing us the biochemical mechanisms that shed even more light on the subject—pardon the pun. Research is finding that even the effectiveness of pharmaceutical medication and chemotherapy drugs depends on what time of day they are given.

Experientially, anyone who travels from one time zone to another understands the importance of circadian rhythm. When your biological timing is severely out of sync with the sun, we call it jet lag. You might not be as sharp as usual, have low energy, have trouble sleeping, and be more prone to getting sick. Fundamentally, jet lag is the blatant recognition that your body's internal clock is on a different schedule than the light and dark cycle of your physical location. Your body is still trying to predict the light cycle from where you departed. Depending on your latitude, the light cycle normally shifts by only a few minutes per day, as the seasons turn. But if you fly and land in a new place on the planet, the light cycle may suddenly and sometimes radically shift. Fortunately, after a few days, your body starts to recalibrate its physiology and gene expression to a rhythm that matches the timing of your new lighting environment. It is estimated that, on average, it takes approximately one day for every hour of time zone difference to recalibrate your natural cycle. So if you travel from London to New York, it will take approximately five days before your body's epigenetic expression will fully adjust to the light cycle of New York.

If you have a circadian mismatch between your body clocks and the natural day/night cycle, it may significantly contribute to the development of any chronic condition and also hinder your ability to recover from any illness. The World Health Organization and other scientific organizations are now classifying nighttime shift work as a probable carcinogen and risk factor for heart disease. And it has been thoroughly documented that swing shift and evening workers have a significant increased risk of all diseases.

OPTIMIZING CIRCADIAN RHYTHM AND SLEEP: LIGHT, HORMONES, AND YOUR BODY'S CLOCK

What is emerging from the research on circadian rhythm is the idea that every cell in your body has an internal clock, and that cell is being guided and entrained by 24-hour circadian rhythms. These cellular clocks are set by the combinatory expression of circadian genes identified as: clock, period, BMAL1, and cryptochrome. Based on repeated daily environmental signals, these internal clocks are set to anticipate events so the cell or organ can "get ready" in advance by initiating the epigenetic expressions ahead of the expected changes coming. This reliable anticipation is based on a number of consistent entrainment cues that primarily include light, temperature, physical activity, and food. And by far the most meaningful influence is light and its corresponding darkness.

As your skin and eyes sense the shift in color and light intensity, they send signals to the internal organs and systems that respond accordingly. In this way, we see how environmental energies affect epigenetic expression. The most prominent mechanism for the body to tell time operates via the eyes. As light enters the eye, photoreceptors detect amazingly subtle shifts in color and intensity of the daylight. Precise information is sent along neural pathways to a tiny region of the brain called the suprachiasmatic nucleus (SCN). This is thought to be your body's master clock. The SCN sends neural signals to parts of the brain called the hypothalamus and pituitary glands.

Why is this important? Essentially, your daily exposure to light and dark is heavily influencing melatonin production, cortisol patterns, thyroid hormone levels, human growth hormone, prolactin, estrogen, testosterone, progesterone, antidiuretic hormone, follicle stimulating hormone, among others. These hormones have a huge impact on a multitude of functions at the cellular and organ level. Ghrelin and leptin, two hormones that are intimately linked with food intake and body weight, are dramatically influenced by light, dark, and sleep.

Studies have shown that, compared with reading a book, just one hour of reading on an electronic device before bed reduces your peak melatonin by about half and delays the peak by two to three hours. Practically, this delays the onset of sleep and significantly diminishes restorative sleep. And when it comes to longevity, melatonin is a pretty important hormone. In addition to initiating sleep, melatonin increases cell regeneration, protects mitochondria by scavenging free radicals, increases glutathione production, and primes the immune system, among other things. Melatonin might just be the longevity king of the hormone world.

Our circadian-rhythm challenges began as society began to live and work almost exclusively indoors, and it has really accelerated in the past 40 years with the advancement of the Internet and computers. As a child, I recall the warnings for watching more than a couple hours of TV each day. With the explosion of computers, phones, and tablets in recent decades, many of us end up staring at extremely bright screens from less than two feet away for more than eight hours each day in our work, school, and social environments. The spectrum of light emitted from phones, TVs, tablets, and computer screens is very, very different from the light emitted by the sun, fire, moon, and stars. And this is especially problematic at night. These artificial spectrums of light have profound effects, stimulating biological functions in ways that we are only beginning to understand.

Circadian rhythm is a critical lifestyle factor that must be optimized in order to generate coherence in the whole body. Not only do your cellular clocks receive light-related signals from the SCN master clock in your brain, but they are also receiving other circadian signals generated by physical activity, food, temperature, and light on the skin. The timing of nearly all biological function is downstream of these environmental queues. If your environment and behavior are consistently synchronized with the daily light and dark cycles, your body will operate in harmony and have the ability to accurately anticipate the timing of appropriate epigenetic signaling tomorrow.

What this all boils down to is that we need to expose our eyes and skin to the daylight when the sun is up and welcome the darkness when the sun is down. It means there are optimal times for activity and other times for rest. There are times when your body is more primed to digest food and other times for fasting. The temperature fluctuations your body experiences should track with Earth's natural 24-hour rhythm—a little warmer during the day and cooler at night. When this occurs, every cell, tissue, and organ will function in greater harmony and exhibit more coherence, resulting in improved operational efficiency and less damage to all systems.

WHEN YOU SLEEP IS AS IMPORTANT AS HOW LONG

Perhaps just as important as how long you sleep is *when* you sleep. Sleeping from midnight to 8 A.M. won't provide you with optimal sleep and recovery, despite getting the recommended seven to nine hours. There are critical sleep windows earlier in the night when most of the deep and restorative sleep takes place and internal cleansing occurs. During this time, the liver is also actively transforming and cleansing the body of the daytime digestive and metabolic activity. But if you're not sleeping during these hours, a wrench is thrown in your biological clockwork and metabolic chaos ensues.

When I asked 35-year-old Javier Armijo of Costa Rica about his parents' way of life, he said, "They didn't have electricity, man, so literally the sun set and that's it for the day. They needed to blow the candle out and go to bed because very early in the morning Grandpa will just wake them up to go work the field." Sixty-eight year-old Cristina Castillo, also from Costa Rica, told me that when she was young, they would all go to sleep around 7 or 8 P.M. to get up at sunrise for work. And 97-year-old Okinawan resident Misako Kamida followed a similar schedule. "I would wake up with the first cuckoo's cry, prepare food, and when it would become brighter outside, start working in the fields. That sort of living has completely transformed now," she said. Similar stories were repeated by elders around the world: they rose with the sun, or just prior, and went to bed a couple hours after sunset at the latest. On average, they would sleep from 9 P.M. to 5 A.M., depending on the season and when the sun set. Their biology was operating on a proper circadian rhythm that slowly adapted as the seasons and light cycles changed. Their days were consistent. They got up at the same time of day and went to bed at the same time each night. Their biology was easily able to anticipate function because they were accustomed and patterned to a typical day.

Unfortunately, most people in the industrialized world have no idea when they should naturally go to bed or wake up. In addition to artificial light, alarm clocks have also played a role in completely dismantling natural sleeping patterns. A loose rule of thumb would be to aim for sleeping from 9 or 10 P.M. to 5 or 6 A.M. However, the more appropriate objective is to let the day and night cycle guide your bedtime and waketime. Everybody has their own inherent sleep schedule that is guided by their genes and entrained by light. Some people are genetic early birds, some are genetic night owls, and some are in the middle. But if your inherited sleep pattern is not properly entrained by the light and dark, you might think you're a night owl when, in fact, you're an early bird.

The key is to let the light and dark cycle of your geographic location set your sleep pattern. Then you must listen to your body. Remember, your body and brain work to anticipate the rhythm of the day and night. So, the more consistency you can create with respect to your sleep time and wake time, the better you will entrain your body's biological rhythms to anticipate function throughout the day and night. This may be challenging at first, but over a couple weeks, this will result in naturally getting tired at the same time of night and getting better quality sleep.

YOUR OPTIMAL EVENING ROUTINE

Imagine what your evenings would be like if you were camping in the wild without electricity, battery-powered lanterns, or your phone. Once the sun set, you only have the moon, stars, and a fire to give you light. When researchers applied this concept in controlled studies, the subjects ended up going to bed two hours earlier than their normal bedtime at home—not because they were bored, but specifically because their biological rhythms began to harmonize with the light cycle and they got tired earlier. One of the biggest opportunities we have to improve circadian rhythm and sleep is to modify our evening routine, and there are a handful of factors to consider.

Reduce Blue and Green Light

The elders lived most of their lives in an environment that had virtually no artificial light. They didn't have to navigate the same obstacles as those of us who live in industrialized societies. Without artificial light, their eyes were able to appropriately sense the color and intensity shifts of the sun's light as it rose in the morning and set in the evening. As the sun sets, the light intensity and amount of natural UV, blue, and green light decrease. Your eyes translate this light information back to your brain's master clock, initiating all the body's nighttime programs, the rise of melatonin, and onset of sleep. In the morning, increasing UV, blue, and green light act as primary signals to your brain that it is daytime. Cortisol rises, melatonin is suppressed, and all the morning epigenetic signals are sent.

Problems tend to arise when your brain and body sense light from artificial sources after the sun has set. Your body has trouble shifting into proper nighttime operation due to excessive emissions of blue and green spectrums of light in particular. One of the most effective ways to help induce sleep onset is to wear blue-light-blocking glasses to filter this light at night. If you struggle with sleep, regular use of blue-light-blocking glasses is a must. Some premium brands do a great job of blocking all the blue and green light, while cheaper brands may only block some of the blue light. If you want better sleep, make sure you're blocking as much blue and green light as possible.

Another important strategy is to reduce the blue- and green-light output from any electronic screens you use after the sun sets. There are several blue-light reduction software and app options that you can download for your electronic devices. The free F.lux product was the first to make a splash, and software like this is well worth installing on as many devices as possible. There are also hardware options that you can purchase to reduce blue light emitted from your TV at night.

Another way to reduce blue and green light is to swap out some overhead lights with blue-free light bulbs from companies like Soraa. Or alternatively, you can scatter a few lamps around the house that only use blue-free light bulbs or orange and red light bulbs. Then you can turn your regular lights off at night and only use the lamps. This creates a pleasantly calm setting that benefits everyone in the space. In the same vein, candles and fire are the best option for sleep and are perhaps even more calming.

If you consistently inhibit blue and green light after the sun sets, your brain and body will slowly recalibrate to your natural sleep rhythm, and you'll more likely start getting tired sometime between 8 and 10 P.M.

Limit Food Consumption within Three Hours of Sleep

Food is another major factor that often flies under the radar when it comes to sleep quality. Eating after sunset is in complete opposition to the normal functional rhythms of the digestive tract, nervous system, and hormonal systems. Research has demonstrated that natural insulin and IGF-1 spikes that occur after a meal will act to reset circadian clock gene expression, disrupting normal sleep patterns. Digestion requires a ton of energetic resource and involves sending a lot of blood to your core, elevating your core body temperature and sending the wrong circadian cues to your body. Not only does eating before bed throw off sleeping patterns, it can hinder your ability to properly digest what you ate because the body's natural rhythm is to shunt energy away from the core at night.

According to 91-year-old Costa Rican Jose Santos, "Dinner was always at five in the afternoon." Do your best to eliminate eating or drinking anything after 7 P.M. or about three hours before bed. This gives your body time to digest the last meal before sleep, so it can dedicate energy to the programs necessary for cleanup, repair, and rejuvenation.

For those who have severe blood sugar issues or insulin resistance, it may be helpful to eat a very small, easily digestible snack about an hour before bed. This will prevent cortisol from rising in an effort to stabilize blood sugar levels. A little warm milk or some nut milk can be good options. With proper circadian rhythm entrainment and other healthy lifestyle habits, blood sugar control will improve over time, allowing you to move away from snacking before bed.

Calm Your Nervous System

A common factor that keeps many people awake in the United States is an overactive mind. It can be a challenge to slow things down in the evening when you have children, work, and spouses to tend to. Social media, news, and politics have a tendency to trigger stress hormones, increase blood pressure, and activate the mind. A busy schedule the next day and a general feeling of overwhelm can keep the mind racing, making it difficult to relax. And if you are dreading your day tomorrow, you may even be subconsciously sabotaging your sleep by staying up later in an attempt to extend the evening and delay the onset of the next day. Or perhaps you've had a fight with or are chronically unhappy with your sleeping partner.

There are many reasons mental/emotional overwhelm can find its way into bed. And all of them shift the balance of the nervous system from the parasympathetic state of rest and digest to the sympathetic state of fight or flight. Hormone cascades radically alter circadian gene expression and sleep patterns, making it very difficult to get a quality night's rest. There are many tools to overcome these obstacles, but first it helps to bring awareness to the issue at hand. Recognize that in the evening, your brain and body want to slow things down. If you don't consistently follow suit, your health will undoubtedly suffer due to the incoherence and disharmony of the nervous system.

If you're overwhelmed with tasks, make a to-do list for the next day. It will ease your mind to get it all on paper. Writing in a journal is another great option. Just write whatever comes to mind or make a list of things you're grateful for. Going for an evening walk after dinner is another great way to let things go. The simple act of light physical movement, fresh air, and nature will calm the nervous system. Reading a real book under blue-free light is another good option. If you're able to do so, taking an Epsom salt bath is an excellent solution to quiet the system and turn down the energetic noise.

One of the most effective ways to activate the parasympathetic nervous system is to use what is known as the calming breath or 4-7-8 breath. It is performed by inhaling through the nose for the count of four, holding for seven seconds, and then releasing out the mouth for eight seconds, making a "whoosh" sound as you release. You should aim to repeat at least five times, but it can be repeated as many times as you like. This breath should be done at least once a day in the evening, but if you can do it more than once a day, you'll certainly benefit from its effects. The greatest benefits will be noticed over time if used with regularity as you are consciously inducing a calming effect on your nervous system with your breath.

Other great options to move and balance your energy include qigong, meditation, or a few restorative yoga poses such as the legs-up-the-wall pose. Whatever methods you choose to incorporate, do your best to create an evening routine that you can sink into and allow your body and mind to become familiar with.

SLEEP HYGIENE

The ambient glow of a bright white street light seeps through window dressings into the bedroom. LED status lights on monitors, televisions, cable boxes, and electronic appliances shine in every room of the house. Digital alarm clocks on bedside nightstands illuminate the room. Central heating keeps the house at a toasty 70 degrees Fahrenheit. And according to a massive body of research, all are working in concert to significantly suppress melatonin production, shorten total sleep time, and dismantle sleep cycles.

Keep It Dark

One of the easiest and most effective strategies for cleaning up your sleep environment is eliminating the light pollution filling your bedroom. Even the seemingly insignificant light sources such as white, blue, or green LED status lights on electronics can slightly disturb sleep.

- If you can, remove objects with status lights from the room all together. Otherwise, you can place black electrical tape over them or purchase inexpensive black-out stickers to place over the lights.

- If you have an electronic clock in your room, it is best to turn off the light or dim it as much as possible.

- Light from the street or nearby houses may be leaking in through your windows as well. If so, blackout curtains will go a long way to creating a more restful sleeping environment.

Once you start eliminating all the small sources of light, you might be amazed at how dark your room can get. The closer you can get to a pitch-black room, the better off your sleep will be.

Minimize EMF Radiation

Visible light isn't the only element that disrupts your sleep environment. Research continues to show that nonvisible light in the form of man-made EMF radiation from mobile phones, Wi-Fi routers, and Bluetooth alters the function of voltage-gated calcium channels at the cellular level, lowering melatonin production and reducing sleep quality. Anybody living in a densely populated, industrialized city is constantly being bathed in an exponentially increasing sea of sleep-disrupting radiation. Unfortunately, for most people, there is no easy way to escape this milieu, although there are reasonable steps you can take to reduce the impact of EMF radiation in your home.

- Before going to bed, turn off your phone or place it in airplane mode. Keeping your phone on, sitting on the night stand next to your head is a sure-fire way to keep you from gaining the full benefits of sleep.

- Another major opportunity to reduce EMF radiation comes from turning off your Wi-Fi router before bed. This can be done manually or with the use of an automated timer that will turn the Wi-Fi router on and off at the time you set.

- If you have the capacity to do so, it can be extremely effective to turn off the electrical breakers in your bedroom or even the whole house.

- If you must keep mobile phones and other devices on that emit EMF, Bluetooth, or mobile signals, keep them as far away from your body as possible. Distance is the most important aspect of reducing the effect of EMF on your biology.

The more you can eliminate electrical fields and EMF radiation, the more likely you are to get a better night's sleep.

Keep It Cool

Throughout the course of history, humans have adapted to the rhythmic temperature fluctuations of the day. We have evolutionarily adapted to higher temperatures during the daytime and lower temperatures after the sun goes down. This decline in environmental temperature helps cue the onset of sleep.

Research shows the brain needs to drop its temperature by about two degrees Fahrenheit to initiate sleep. And due to the body's natural rhythms and resource allocation, core body temperature also begins to decrease in the afternoon in preparation for sleep. From your peak afternoon core body temperature to the lowest point just prior to waking up, core body temperature will drop about two degrees Fahrenheit as well.

During REM sleep, your brain temperature rises and your ability to thermoregulate body temperature slightly declines. In this phase of sleep, your body temperature is more heavily influenced by the temperature of the environment. Conversely, during non-REM sleep, your brain and body temperature tend to fall together. If your core body temperature is unable to remain low, your sleep will suffer.

Creating a relatively cool sleep environment will help induce deeper sleep and assist with sleep onset. Try setting the thermostat somewhere between 62 and 67 degrees Fahrenheit at 8 or 9 P.M. to help induce drowsiness as you get ready for bed.

Another strategy you can use to lower your core body temperature is to have a light sauna or take a hot shower or bath before bed. Paradoxically you will feel nice and warm when you're done. But because blood is moving from the core to the surface, you'll actually be radiating heat out of your body.

Sleep Orientation

Most individuals have a preferred sleeping position, whether it is left side, right side, back, or stomach. According to both modern science and Ayurveda, sleeping position matters. Ayurvedic wisdom and modern scientific research both suggest the best sleeping position for most people is on their left side, with the left ear on the pillow. This is said to aid digestion and improve lymphatic drainage.

According to Ayurveda, some people will benefit from sleeping on their right side. If you have a more active, fiery, competitive, and driven energy (pitta type), sleeping on your right side may help cool and calm your system as a result of breathing primarily through the left nostril.

Ayurvedic wisdom suggests that sleeping on your back is generally not the best for most people, but if your head is supported correctly and your breathing is not obstructed, it can be okay for some.

Sleeping on your stomach is generally considered the worst position by both Ayurveda and most scientific findings. Not only does this position restrict breathing and place added pressure on your internal organs, but your neck and spine are also not well-supported or properly aligned.

No matter which sleeping position you choose, it is well documented that mouth breathing during sleep is detrimental to your health. Mouth breathing can negatively impact dental health; immune function; create an imbalance of CO_2 and oxygen in the body; impair your parasympathetic tone; reduce nitric oxide in the blood; and disrupt restorative sleep cycles. Conversely, breathing through your nose increases parasympathetic response, increases deep sleep, and improves overall health. If you are a mouth breather, you can experiment with different sleeping positions and use specialized mouth tape to help keep your mouth closed, prevent snoring, and facilitate nose breathing during sleep.

According to Ayurveda, the direction in which you sleep also matters. To quote one of the greatest, living Ayurvedic masters, Dr. Vasant Lad, "Only dead people sleep pointing north." It is said that sleeping with your head pointing north draws energy out of the body. The magnetic polarity of the body is such that your head is the positive pole and your feet the negative. If you sleep with your head facing north, you'll have two positive poles in the same direction, which disturbs blood circulation and digestion and increases stress in the body.

Sleeping with your head to the west is also ill-advised. While not as disruptive as north, it is said that sleeping with your head to the west will decrease deep sleep, increase active dreaming, and increase ambition in life.

Sleeping with your head pointing east is said to be ideal for students as it increases memory, creativity, and concentration, and improves meditation or other spiritual pursuits.

According to Ayurveda, sleeping with your head pointing south is the most optimal direction to sleep as it promotes deep, restorative sleep, improving overall health and well-being. While this all may sound like folk wisdom, scientific studies have recently discovered that humans have a magnetic sense that allows the brain to detect the Earth's magnetic field. So perhaps there is something to this ancient wisdom. It is certainly worth experimenting!

DAILY ROUTINE

The other side of the sleep and circadian rhythm equation that is often neglected is the morning after. If you're being woken up by a sudden stimulus in the form of noise, light, or movement, it's safe to say you could be getting better sleep. Using an alarm clock to wake up every day is one of the major causes of sleep deprivation. And when you're woken up in the middle of Stage 3 or 4 deep sleep, you probably feel extremely groggy.

If the body wants to sleep, you really should let it sleep. The modern world carries with it significant challenges here as most people have a set time they need to wake up. Whether it's a long commute to work, or getting the kids ready for school, or getting to work before the stock market opens, there are plenty of inflexible situations that require an alarm clock. The way to overcome this is to do whatever you can to get to bed early enough to get your required sleep. As much as possible, continue to push your bedtime earlier until you wake up before your alarm. In order to initiate drowsiness earlier in the evening, you may have to really focus on avoiding blue and green light as early as possible.

The other aspect of sleep that you might be able to work into your day is an afternoon nap. Research shows that sleep patterns associated with normal circadian rhythms will often include a period in the afternoon where the sleep urge spikes before coming back down. This asymmetrical sleep pattern is quite normal and is something most of the elders followed. Commonly known as a *siesta*, they frequently took naps after lunch, when the intensity of the sun was peaking. A 30- to 60-minute nap in the afternoon allows the body to catch up considerably on sleep without significantly disrupting evening sleeping patterns.

Other than an afternoon nap, there are a number of strategies and methods you can use throughout your day to improve sleep at night. The more you can synchronize your behavior with the daily cycle and expose your eyes to natural light, the more you set the tone for good sleep at night.

Jump-Start Your Engine

If your morning cortisol is chronically low or you simply have low energy when you wake up, there are two excellent methods you can use within the first 30 minutes of waking to help increase your morning cortisol peak, known as your cortisol awakening response (CAR).

The first option is to perform three to five minutes of a relatively intense exercise. This might include push-ups, pull-ups, lunges, burpees, jump rope, running, or anything else you can think of to get the blood pumping, including sex.

The second method is to use an energizing breathwork technique sometimes called the breath of fire. This is a rapid, rhythmic, and continuous breath done through the nostrils with the mouth closed. The pace is typically two to three cycles per second with equal inhale and exhale. This stimulating technique helps synchronize the biorhythms of all the body's systems; improves the balance between the sympathetic and parasympathetic nervous systems; and improves circulation and detoxification. Due to its ability to stimulate your system, there are some contraindication to be mindful of. It is best not to practice this breath if you are pregnant; have high blood pressure or heart issues; vertigo; spinal issues; or a respiratory issue. It is always best to consult your health-care provider if you have any concerns.

Expose Your Eyes to the Daylight

One of the most effective strategies you can use to entrain your circadian rhythm and improve sleep at night is to expose your eyes to sunlight first thing in the morning and as often as possible throughout the day. Light from the sun can be 1,000 times brighter than indoor lighting, and your biology will respond to this powerful signal. For some, increasing daylight in their eyes first thing in the morning can be life-changing.

As soon you are done with the short burst of movement or breathwork upon waking, try going for a 20-minute walk outside. If you're unable to go for a walk, you can just sit outside with a cup of herbal tea for 20 minutes. In order for your master clock to know when the sun comes up, your eyes must get exposed to the daylight. It may seem insignificant, but this doesn't happen to the degree necessary to set the circadian clock in many people. Without sufficient daylight first thing in the morning, there is no strong circadian queue. This lack of light causes cortisol production to suffer during the day and melatonin production to suffer at night. Daylight in your eyes in the morning, coupled with darkness at night, is the best recipe for a strong spike of melatonin, along with quality, restorative sleep.

To a lesser extent, full-spectrum sunlight on the skin can also improve cortisol in the morning and melatonin production at night. Research has found that human skin cells have receptors for both serotonin and melatonin. They can also produce serotonin and convert it to melatonin when exposed to light from the sun. Recently, researchers also discovered that corticotrophin-releasing hormone is produced in the skin in response to sunlight. This is the hormone that initiates cortisol production to help to wake you up and deal with stress. Particularly for those who work indoors, it can be very important to expose as much of your skin as possible to the sun, even in short bouts during the day—so long as you don't burn.

Reduce Caffeine Consumption

This is always the least popular suggestion I have for the clients I work with, but it often surprises them how much of a difference this makes in their overall energy and sleep patterns. For some, caffeine does not have much of a deleterious effect. For others, it can wreak havoc on their system. It's like stealing energy from tomorrow to get through today. Oftentimes, you can't get an accurate gauge until you give it up for at least a week.

Throughout the day, the neurotransmitter adenosine accumulates in your body and brain as a result of normal metabolic activity—specifically, using adenosine triphosphate (ATP). The accumulation of adenosine in the brain and nervous system helps to calm your system down, causing you to feel increasingly tired the longer you are awake. During sleep, adenosine is cleared, allowing you to feel more alert the following day. One of the reasons caffeine can be so problematic for sleep is that it blocks the effects of adenosine on your brain and nervous system, causing you to feel alert when you normally would feel tired.

If you're a big coffee or tea drinker, try first scaling back a bit and take your time weaning off completely. Try switching to herbal teas or coffee alternatives that don't contain caffeine. Most decaf coffee uses harsh chemicals to remove the caffeine, but there are some that use healthier methods. Look for the package to say solvent-free, Swiss-water process, certified organic, or chemical free. If you can't give up the coffee or tea, do your best to limit consumption and don't drink any past noon.

Ditch the Shades

This may seem like a strange recommendation, but this can make a huge difference when it comes to both circadian rhythm entrainment and eye health. The modern version of sunglasses were only invented in 1929. For thousands of years prior, humans walked this earth without sunglasses, using only hats and other garments to shade the sun. In part because they are a fashion accessory, wearing sunglasses outside at all times has become all too common. And it's not a coincidence that today many people have become visually sensitive to sunlight. Fortunately, this can be improved through regular exposure to daylight without the use of sunglasses.

Studies have demonstrated that natural light actually has a positive role to play when it comes to eye health. Myopia or nearsightedness has exploded over the past 50 years. What researchers have found is that children who spend more time outside develop myopia at a far lesser rate than their peers who spend less time outside. Neither 92-year-old Marta Congia of Sardinia nor 97-year-old Hideko Kamida of Okinawa wore sunglasses over the course of their lives. And neither of them require reading glasses at their age. In fact, Hideko Kamida was barefoot reading the paper when we visited.

The various colors and frequencies in sunlight serve an important role as they carry information to the brain via intrinsically photosensitive retinal ganglion cells (ipRGCs). By altering the light frequencies with sunglasses, you're sending a fraudulent message to your brain about the environment. Regular safe exposure of your eyes to daylight—even on a cloudy day, and perhaps with a hat—may help improve your circadian biology and better maintain your vision as you get older.

THE GREAT OUTDOORS

As I flew from the busy metropolis of Athens to learn about the ways of the elders on the island of Ikaria, the sudden contrast of the two Greek landscapes was shocking. One of my favorite aspects of Athens is the busy nightlife and late-night dining in the old town. With flavors of New York City, Athens is vibrant and full of energy. In the summer after 9 P.M., the locals and tourists gather to dine in the streets. But as soon as we touched down on the tiny island of Ikaria, the evening was silent and dark. The main tourist area was quiet with only a few diners scattered about the few late-night restaurants.

Other than the main port, Ikaria is comprised of small village centers and rural living. It felt like I was instantly transported back in time. Commerce was primarily carried out by mom-and-pop shops and small markets that only operated during the day. The lack of evening activity and nominal automobile traffic established no need for street lighting in most areas. The night sky was dark blue, lighted only by the half moon and a million stars. I felt small and insignificant gazing at the heavens above.

With the significant lack of infrastructure, I was prompted to ask 90-year-old Yannoula Kratzas when electricity was first used in town. "They brought electricity to Pera Arethousa village in 1978, but they didn't bring it to our place. Before that we were using carbide lamps at night while knitting and mending clothes or telling stories," she replied. Similar anecdotes were told by the elders in Sardinia, Costa Rica, and Okinawa as well. The installation of an electrical grid had only come into existence in the rural areas in the past 30 years or so. Virgilio Angulo of Nicoya, Costa Rica, told me, "The first block of electric energy came in 1950. But before that, we used gas on the street corner, lit by a lamplighter to give light in the street." And this was in the second largest town on the peninsula. In each of the four longevity regions around the world, the elders lived most of their lives only having a few dimly lit gas lamps and maybe a fireplace as their source of evening light. Contrast that to today in the same region of Nicoya, Virgilio said, "Well, this is a completely different phase of life. A child nowadays comparatively to a child 25 years ago, it's not even remotely the same. Now everything is Internet, computer, telephones. And this all started around twenty years ago."

As modern culture has pushed forth with greater technological advancement, even in these remote towns, it seems as though there has been a growing perception that humanity is separate from nature—perhaps even superior. But humanity's greatest ills are created when our perceptions are in opposition to nature's truths.

For thousands of years of recorded human history, light only came from a few sources—the moon, stars, sun, fire, and lightning. That radically changed when Thomas Edison commercialized the light bulb in 1879 and sparked perhaps the most significant change to our environment in recorded history. The widespread use of electricity was undoubtedly the single biggest driver of economic growth and increased comfort the world has ever seen. For this reason, we wisely welcomed it with open arms. Electricity has been the lifeblood of nearly everything that has contributed to greater health and longer life in the 20th century. It also began a relatively quick path to one of the biggest silent disrupters of human health, as widespread use of artificial light has become the lynchpin for our near complete isolation from the natural world.

A recent poll conducted by a laundry detergent company in the United Kingdom found that 20 percent of children did not play outside at all on an average day. Of the 12,000 parents surveyed across 10 countries, they found that $1/3$ of children ages 5 to 12 spend less than 30 minutes outside each day. While this is not a scientific study, it aligns with an official, two-year government study in the United Kingdom that found that 12 percent of English children had never visited a natural environment (e.g. park, forest, beach) in the previous year. A 2012 study of U.S. preschool-age children showed similar results. Half of the 8,950 children in the study did not have even one supervised outdoor play opportunity with a parent per day on average.

By insulating ourselves from the natural world, we lose touch with the heartbeat of the Earth, known as the Schumann resonance. We aren't able to freely exchange electric charges between our feet and the bare earth. We lose touch with beneficial environmental microbes that educate and improve our immune system. We don't take advantage of the health benefits of fluctuating temperatures. And we shield ourselves from the ultimate source of life on this planet—the sun. All of which is in complete opposition to how the elders were raised. They were more in touch with the Earth both physically and energetically. They slept lower to the ground. They walked barefoot. These simple habits gave them a more intimate relationship with nature.

In Costa Rica, Cristina Castillo and her family did so with intention. "My father said that to walk on the ground was to raise our defenses (build immunity). And he always told us that. He never gave us the opportunity to wear shoes. We all walked to create defenses. We would take a little kid to the ocean and bathe them there so he wouldn't suffer from colds—from all the iodine in the ocean. And that was it. We never worried about bacteria." Almost all their life was spent outside when they were young. Even when we visited, most people were outside when they were home. Or they were in an open-air environment, exposed to the elements. And one thing's for sure, they had absolutely no fear about the sun. Jose Santos was 91 years old when we chatted, and he told me, "We used to work from sunrise to sunset. Nobody blocked the sunlight. Our hat protected us."

Life in the modern world can now be lived almost exclusively devoid of the outdoors. Many people in urban areas go days or weeks without touching their bare feet to the earth, especially when the weather is unfavorable. We put our shoes on before we leave the house, drive to work, spend eight hours in an office, drive home, and finish the evening inside our comfortable homes. This is a dramatic shift from the intimate connection with nature for nearly all human history. There are countless reasons to spend more time outside, but a few are really worth highlighting.

Heliotherapy and Your Hormones

The sun is the source of all life on this planet. Exposure to sunlight is a vital requirement, yet we've been conditioned to fear it. There is no question that excessive UV radiation can cause DNA damage, leading to cancer and visible aging of the skin. But there are tremendous benefits that full-spectrum sunlight provides, so it is important to get appropriate doses on your skin.

Your skin is packed full of light receptors called chromophores that store photonic energy from the sun. Amino acids like tryptophan, tyrosine, phenylalanine, and histidine along with urocanic acid and nucleic acids and many others deep in the skin all absorb light from the sun. Termed photoendocrinology, your ability to capture light in the skin has massive implications on your body's hormonal systems. If you don't get enough sunlight on the skin, you're likely to experience suboptimal hormone and neurotransmitter function that affect your body composition, sex drive, energy status, sleep, immune system, and mood.

Healthy and balanced function requires a certain amount of natural sunlight on your skin and in your eyes to initiate entire cascades of function in the body. The production of vitamin D, which is really a hormone, is of course critical for immune function and building healthy bone structure. Light from the sun also works with cholesterol in your skin to produce testosterone, progesterone, and growth hormones. The skin is the body's largest organ and serves as the interface between the outer world and our internal biology. If we spend 95 percent of our time inside, we're missing large doses of light that our biology has been accustomed to receiving for thousands of years—most notably UV and infrared light.

Follow the Seasons to Minimize Sun Damage

It is interesting to note that the elders we visited never used chemical sun creams to block the sun, even after it became available to them. They were regularly exposed to full-spectrum sunlight. However, the elders weren't lying out on a beach getting a tan; they were working outside and interacting with their environment. They also shielded during the hottest times of the day, often taking a one- or two-hour siesta in the shade.

Our relationship with the sun in the 21st century has been skewed by both commercial advertising and mainstream medical voices. The pain of sunburns coupled with the risk of skin cancer has created an unhealthy fear of the sun. However, there is a lot of research that supports the healing benefits of sunlight. If we learn to better harmonize with the seasons, optimize our circadian rhythm, get good sleep, eat real food, avoid petrochemicals, and avoid sunburns, skin cancer would be quite rare. The objective should be to get sun on your skin while avoiding the damage of burning. If you can view sunlight, in the right dose, as a carrier of medicine, it may be just that for you.

When determining the right amount of sun exposure for you, it is important to be mindful of the interaction between your heritage, your skin color, and your geography. For example, if you have the red hair and fair skin of your Irish ancestors and live under the intense rays of Australia, you will burn and experience sun damage quickly. On the other end of the spectrum, if you have dark skin and live in a northern climate, you may actually *require* more time in the sun to get the benefits and maintain a healthy balance of function. Keep the following guidelines in mind:

- Expose your skin to the morning and late afternoon sun only.

- Avoid the sun midday as much as possible.

- Spend more time in the winter sun. Decrease your time during the spring, and decrease it even more in the summer. Slowly increase with the autumn sun in a repeating cycle, season after season and year after year.

- The best option for sun protection is clothing, a hat, and shade cover.

- If you must use sun cream, choose zinc oxide over other chemical blockers. You can check with the Environmental Working Group to find a list of the safest brands.

I don't recommend most commercial sunblocks, as they contain harsh chemicals that can accumulate in the body and create a lot of health challenges over time. The other main issue with sun creams is that most of them will do a good job of blocking UVB, thus saving you from damaging rays and a sunburn. But they do a poor job of blocking UVA, giving you a false sense of security since excessive UVA light can also cause DNA and skin damage. Be wary of zinc nanoparticle sun creams. They not only have the ability to cross the blood-brain-barrier, they also tend to be damaging to sea life.

If you're able to bring awareness to your body's natural rhythms and create alignment with the sun's daily and seasonal rhythm where you live, you'll likely notice a dramatic improvement in the way you look, think, feel, and sleep. Understanding and applying the general concepts of sleep, circadian rhythm, and light may be the most impactful piece to the longevity puzzle for many people. You can be eating the right foods and doing all the right exercises, but if you're doing it at the wrong time, you're still going to be creating disharmony as your brain and body work unnecessarily hard to maintain homeostasis. If you flow with the rhythms of nature instead of swimming against the current, you'll find that everything else you're doing to improve your health will have a much greater effect.

Chapter 5

EAT TO THRIVE

In food is excellent medicine, in food is bad medicine;
good and bad are relative.

— TRANSLATION FROM THE TEXT *DE ALIMENTO*,
COMMONLY ATTRIBUTED TO HIPPOCRATES

For most us who live in a culture that has an overabundance of food options, choosing an appropriate diet might just be the most confusing and challenging aspect of healthy living. In the book *The Paradox of Choice* by Barry Schwartz, the author details the psychological, emotional, and lifestyle implications of having a great deal of options when trying to make a decision. In short, choice overload tends to increase mental and emotional stress. The more choices we have, the more confusing things get and the harder it is to make a correct and informed choice. Thus, the harder it is to feel confident you're making the *best* choice.

Dietary theory in the Western world over the past hundred years has been a fascinating roller coaster of ideas, beliefs, and scientific back and forth. All the doctors, nutritionists, and health experts I know are all doing their best to share the healthiest and most accurate information with respect to diet. Yet the recommendations vary wildly! Today, with a variety of popular diets, food has easily become a central topic of debate in the health world.

There are even attempts to identify a single dietary strategy that will universally lead to optimal health and longevity.

So how can we make sense of this topic of food—something so fundamental to our existence? The truth is, each one of the whole-foods based dietary strategies stands on solid scientific ground. But also, there is no diet that works for everyone. Rather, we all have our own unique constitution to consider and a number of lifestyle factors that create context around the types of food that may be best for each individual. That said, there is a way to navigate the waters, and there are certainly a number of dietary principles that are universal to human health. While modern science is helpful, I learned a lot more about food from chatting with the elders around the world.

LESSONS FROM THE ELDERS

In examining the diets of the various elders around the world, one thing stood out above all else—balance. There were no secrets, special foods, or strict rules that equated to health. They all ate in a way that made sense based on their geography, season, and circumstance.

All the elders ate a notably distinct diet from one another, and each culture shared only a few foods in common. But what remained consistent were the dietary philosophies. Meals were almost always communal, shared with family and friends. In fact, we often got invited for a meal with the extended family after we were done filming interviews with locals. Preparing the food was a group activity, and they did not rush through their meals, as it was a time to relax and connect with all who were present. Almost all their food came from the backyard garden or a small plot nearby, depending on what was in season. None of their diets could be classified as any of the popular dietary approaches today. The elders from Ikaria and Sardinia could generally be classified as following the endlessly studied Mediterranean diet. But the elders from Guanacaste and Okinawa follow very different dietary frameworks.

Growing up in agrarian villages, the elders primarily ate plant foods throughout their life because it could be inexpensively grown and harvested most of the year. They'd harvest wild fruits, roots, tubers, and vegetables in season. Meat was consumed far less often and in much lower quantities than we typically see in Western cultures. Because the elders spent most of their life without refrigeration, meat required more resources to raise, buy, and preserve. As such, meat was eaten sporadically or generally when they could be afforded. In each location, it was typical to hunt wild game and raise pigs, chickens, goats, or cows. They often collected eggs from the hens they raised. Milk, cheese, and yogurt were produced from the cows, goats, or sheep raised on their property.

According to everyone I spoke with across the cultures, their diets consisted largely of complex carbohydrates and starches such as wheat, rice, potatoes, beans, squash, and root vegetables. Leafy salads were quite uncommon as we have come to know them in the West. And if we try to imagine what life was like without electricity, having to grow most of your own food, it makes sense that leafy greens were not a staple. They wanted to grow foods that contained a lot of caloric energy and would satiate them and their families. Large amounts of leafy greens, as healthy as they are, just didn't provide the sustenance they needed.

They all lived off the land according to their cultural influence. When the food you grow and the animals you raise or hunt are your only sources of food, there is little room for discrimination or extreme dietary philosophies. They simply didn't have the luxury to choose a dietary approach beyond what nature afforded them. It was all too common to experience minor bouts of food shortage, crop decimation due to weather, and severe economic challenges. At the same time, they didn't have to deal with "the paradox of choice" either. Each of them seemed to be very in tune with what personally served them well in the context of their environment, and they all ate according to their preferences without any staunch rules.

In analyzing the cultural diets described by the elders around the world, there are a few common variables:

1. Their diets consisted of organic, whole foods that were minimally processed.

2. Staples consisted of one or more of the following: rice, beans, legumes, potatoes, corn.

3. Diets were primarily, but not exclusively, plant-based, with plenty of starchy carbohydrates and vegetables with occasional meat.

4. Foods were eaten in season and usually homegrown, foraged, or locally sourced.

So-Called Problematic Foods

What was perhaps most fascinating to me was how many foods the elders would eat that are commonly thought of as problematic in the West. For example, bread was and still is an absolute staple in the villages of Sardinia. They practically laughed at me when I asked about the potential health issues bread may cause. Sardinian resident Dr. Giovanni Ugas elaborated on its use. "Bread was the fundamental food, because we would always eat bread with everything. If the bread was missing in a house, it was the end of it. So everything could be missing, but not bread. From breakfast on, it accompanied everything else. You wouldn't eat anything without bread. The bread was decorated; it had extraordinary symbolism. So it was connected to everyday life and the holy days. So I repeat, it was formidable and fundamental for nutrition."

In Costa Rica, corn was and still is a staple food, along with rice and beans. When I interviewed Luciano Grijalva in his rural home, he said, "I believe people can attribute longevity to the consumption of corn. Because all the people in Guanacaste consume corn. All the typical foods are derived from corn as a base. And our native people had corn as a base, and those people had longevity too. Here, the majority of people consume corn. If you go to Nicoya, everyone sells corn; tortillas, empanadas, etcetera. Everything is base of corn. I think that maybe that helps lengthen lives." He even had a large, hand-turned, mechanical corn mill in his backyard that he still consistently uses to this day.

When it comes to beans and other legumes, the longevity regions I visited have a long history of eating a diet primarily consisting of lectin-rich foods. Lectins are a class of proteins found in a wide variety of plants and some meats. Labeled "antinutrients" for their ability to bind to carbohydrates and micronutrients, as well as inhibit digestive enzymes, lectins are considered one of the most significant problems in the Western diet by some experts. Recent research, however, demonstrates that a moderate amount of dietary lectins can have cellular antioxidant effects and help stabilize blood sugar. Studies are also looking at using certain lectins in anticancer treatments due to their ability to kill cancer cells.

When I spoke to the three Melis brothers of Sardinia, all over 91 years old at the time, Vitalio Melis said, "We would have minestrone soup everyday for lunch, for dinner always, always. We would race to eat it. It was very good. Of course, made with healthy ingredients, our own olive oil. Anyway, that was our main food." The ingredients in their beloved minestrone soup? Potatoes, beans, chickpeas, lard, cheese, tomato, and a few vegetables. Interestingly, the Melis family is in the *Guinness Book of World Records* for having the oldest combined age of any family ever recorded. In June 2012, the six sisters and three brothers had a combined age of 818 years. Their ages ranged from 89 years old to 105 years old. Sounds like their family was doing something right.

How much fruit you should eat is also something that is debated in the West. You might hear suggestions on limiting fruit intake because it is high in fructose and other sugars. This wasn't a concern with those I spoke with in Costa Rica. When I asked Javier if he and his family ate a lot of fruit, he confirmed, saying, "All the fruits, and not only the ones from supermarket or the fruit stands, but some of the others as well. This place specifically is full of guava, mangos, and another fruit called jocote, a tiny, wild plum."

When I asked if he worried about fruit making him fat because of all the sugar, he responded, perplexed, "No, what do you mean? No."

"That's a perception in the States that people are afraid fruits will make them fat," I said.

"How, because of the sugar? Does sugar make you fat?"

"That's the misconception," I responded.

"No, man," he said, shaking his head with a laugh.

There is value in analyzing the food choices of those who have lived a long life and the dietary cuisines of their culture. But there is a real intellectual danger in assuming that copying their food choices will necessarily translate to good health for you or me. What their collective diets do show us, however, is that it doesn't make sense to classify entire food groups or any specific food as unhealthy for all people. So how do we square this with some of the advice by various experts that may suggest otherwise?

I invite you to open up to the possibility that the experts may have good information that may or may not apply to you, specifically. Because we all have a unique constitution and highly specific lifestyle contexts, what may be absolute truth for one person may be blatantly incorrect for another. I've noticed that health consumers have adopted so many restrictions around food in the past 30 years, resulting in a great deal of anxiety, fear, confusion, and frustration. In order to avoid this, it can be helpful to be open to all dietary information, hold it lightly, and let your body guide you.

CONSIDERING FOOD SENSITIVITIES AND IMMUNE TOLERANCE

There is no question that over the past few decades in the United States, food allergies, sensitivities, and food-related conditions have been on the rise in a big way. The list of common problematic foods is long and seems to be getting longer. The usual culprits include peanuts, wheat, gluten, corn, soy, rice, oats, beans, tree nuts, nightshades, yeast, citrus fruits, eggs, cow dairy, shellfish, caffeine. But more and more people are finding themselves with sensitivities and reactions to what seem like benign foods such as cucumber, avocado, celery, and the list goes on.

In my own practice, it was the norm for my clients to have notable issues with certain foods. And the natural tendency is to look at what ingredient or aspect of the food might be causing the problem. As such, nutrition researchers have identified loads of potential perpetrators. The following is just a small sampling of the compounds in everyday foods that have been identified as problematic: gluten, wheat germ agglutinin, gliadin, glutenin, gluteomorphin, transglutaminase, phytic acid, salicylates, A1 beta-casein, oxalic acid, lectins, fructose, lactose, stachyose, raffinose, yeast, Neu5Gc, purines, histidine, egg proteins.

The scientific research isn't wrong. There are a great many natural food compounds that can create inflammation and activate an immune response given the right conditions. But in my experience, the food itself is usually not the source of the problem.

Analogously, if my house is on fire, and I try to put it out with gasoline, the fire will rage and worsen. But gasoline didn't start the fire—it only aggravated the conditions. If I pour gasoline on my friend's house that isn't on fire, nothing happens. And if I pour gasoline in the tank of my car, it acts as fuel. This is akin to what's happening with our food in the modern world. In most cases of food sensitives, there is inherent damage at the level of the gastrointestinal tract, immune system, or nervous system that leads to imbalanced gut-immune function, excessive inflammation, and hyperpermeability of the gut lining (leaky gut). In essence, the body is on fire and any food can become the gasoline.

The point here is not to suggest you should eat loads of allergens, industrialized sugar products, or any food that might give you issues—quite the opposite. Any food that creates noticeable symptoms or any immune response should be avoided until the GI tract, immune system, or nervous system is healed and gut-immune regulation is balanced. But if we mistake the food for the cause of the issue instead of just the trigger, the core imbalance—GI dysfunction—is likely to be overlooked.

I have seen this situation many times in my practice. A client may have started with eliminating four or five problematic foods. Over time, the list would grow to 10 or 20 problematic foods. Eventually it could get so bad that there could end up being only four or five foods that *don't* cause an inflammatory reaction. This is the danger in thinking that the food is the source of the issue.

Improve Your Immune Tolerance

Gastrointestinal conditions have skyrocketed over the past few decades, and the primary reason is that many in the Western cultures have disconnected from the natural world. We've gotten out of alignment with nature. We've lost coherence. From an immunological perspective, we've lost our tolerance.

Immunological tolerance broadly refers to how your system reacts to the world and whether your regulatory T-cells are going to develop an inflammatory response to the environment. It is the primary mechanism your body uses to identify foreign invaders. Generally speaking, if you have balanced and effective regulatory T-cell function, you're much less likely to react to foods.

Researchers have identified a number of ways to improve immune tolerance. These include sunlight, vitamin D3, fat soluble vitamin A, gut microbiota diversity, movement, diversity of plants in your diet, quality sleep, fasting, blood sugar stability, aligned circadian rhythm, limbic retraining therapy, and natural opioids generated through positive thoughts and emotions. On the flip side, there are a number of things that appear to disrupt immune tolerance, including petrochemicals, excessive pharmaceutical drugs, chemical pesticides, highly processed foods, poor sleep, gastrointestinal infections, excessive mental-emotional stress, vitamin and nutrient deficiencies, and poor digestion of food.

Improving tolerance may take consistency and time, but it is the key to eliminating food sensitivities for good. If you're able to maintain integrity of your gut lining, you're able to properly digest foods, and you maintain good immune tolerance, food sensitivities won't be an issue for you. As it turns out, the elders lived in a way that improved immune tolerance and weren't exposed to the myriad of modern, industrial factors that destroy it.

FOOD IS INFORMATION

It seems scientific research is identifying a new reason each week that some seed, berry, herb, or mushroom is healthy. I'm willing to bet that the more research we do, the more "disease-fighting" compounds and mechanisms we'll find. Beyond the macromolecules such as fats, proteins, and carbohydrates, all the vitamins and minerals are also sending signals to your DNA, altering genetic expression. And beyond those is a whole spectrum of phytochemicals, polyphenols, fibers, beta-glucans, and the like that are also communicating with your DNA.

If you recall from Chapter 1, there is also an intermediate step of communication to this process. As your food enters your GI tract, your microbes are helping to metabolize all these compounds. When they do, they produce secondary metabolites, new molecules that signal to other microbes in your GI tract as well as to your mitochondrial DNA and human DNA. If that wasn't enough, the communication is not unidirectional. Your mitochondrial DNA and human DNA are also communicating with each other and with the microbes you house. That's right—you have food, microbes, mitochondria, and human cells all in communication based on the information that is contained within the food. In our modern age, that information has been changed due to nonorganic foods, GMOs, and heavy commercial processing.

Go Organic

You know what my grandmother called an organic tomato? She called it a tomato. Chemical fertilizers and pesticides are a very new experiment for humanity—and things are not looking good. As it turns out, there is a tremendous price to pay for disrupting the natural biome of food crops as they grow.

The soil environment is probably the most important factor in determining the type of information that your body will receive from the plant and animal foods you consume. Two beets grown in different soils will generally look and taste the same, but the information contained in and on the beets may be wildly different. The soil is an amazingly complex ecosystem in and of itself, and the beet will grow in response to this complex ecosystem. If the soil is healthy, balanced, full of life, and of the correct conditions, the beet will express its genes in harmony with the environment, producing a robust and healthy beet that is capable of withstanding a challenging predatory environment. With the help of symbiotic microorganisms in the soil ecosystem, the beet will adapt by producing polyphenols and a strong phytochemical defense system to protect itself from predation. And it is these phytochemical and polyphenol profiles that act as the plant's immune system. They show up as the red color in beets, the pungent taste in garlic, the green skin of the apple, the brownish red in cacao, and the bitterness in broccoli.

So if your food is grown in beneficial conditions with adequate stress above ground and below the soil, the more likely you are to have a robust phytochemical defense, and the more these compounds can benefit you and your immune system. Unfortunately, it is all too common to have the same crops growing in the same soil year after year with little replenishment. Over time, if enough pesticides, herbicides, and chemical fertilizers are used on the soil, it becomes practically lifeless. If the soil lacks microorganisms, the plant cannot reach its full potential, and its phytochemical defenses won't thoroughly develop—which often necessitates more pesticides and fertilizer. What's more, the plant will likely contain greater levels of chemicals, metals, and other environmental pollutants because the soil is lacking the microorganisms that have the ability to break these things down. While it is often difficult to determine the soil quality of the food you buy, it is important to make sure the food is at least organic. Better yet, if you feel inclined, growing your own food is the surest way to guarantee the healthiest soil and healthiest food.

Another benefit to organic foods that don't get sprayed with chemical fertilizers, pesticides, and cleaning agents has to do with the biome on the food itself. For the elders, it was quite common to pick fruits off trees, vegetables off vines, and roots out of the soil, and give them nothing more than a quick wipe or rinse before eating them. In so doing, they are maintaining a high degree of microbial population and diversity that lives on the exterior of the food. While this may sound trivial, the implications may be quite profound, according to newer research on the human microbiome and immune system.

In order to develop and maintain a robust and adaptive immune system, your body requires frequent interaction with environmental microbes to help modulate and regulate immune function in order to adapt and meet the demands of a changing environment. In a sense, it's like a workout for your immune system.

Avoid GMOs

Another major shift we've seen in the United States over the past 30 years in particular is the use of genetically modified organisms (GMOs). Many of these GMOs have been created by biotech companies so crops will survive even greater pesticide use. If the seeds weren't genetically modified, the toxic pesticides would kill the natural form of the plant. Thirty years of side-by-side studies conducted by the Rodale Institute show that organic crops are just as pest resistant as their GMO counterparts, but the organic crops outperform the GMO crops in times of harsh weather. So there really is no need to genetically modify nature's food supply.

The most prevalent GMO foods include corn, sugar beets, soy, tomatoes, cotton, canola, flax, and Hawaiian papaya. And unfortunately, corn, sugar beets, and soy end up in a large majority of processed food products in one way or another, including meat. Virgilio Angulo of Costa Rica informed me that the fertilizer companies were trying to give away GMO seeds in his village in an attempt to sell them chemical fertilizers. It didn't take, as most of the locals realized the benefits of using organic seeds and natural fertilizers.

Research continues to show that these GMO crops create a leaky gut barrier and significant issues for our gut microbiota, resulting in unfavorable epigenetic expression and elevated inflammation. At very low doses, the chemical pesticides can make their way past the immune system to damage the DNA directly. One study looked at mice that were fed Roundup-ready soybeans for eight months. They developed damage to their liver, pancreas, and testicles. When they were put on a non-GMO soy diet for the next month, these conditions started to reverse. These types of results have also been seen in livestock.

Unfortunately, GMOs are quite ubiquitous in the food supply, particularly in packaged foods. It is difficult to estimate the overall exposure of the average person, but one study in Canada revealed that 91 percent of pregnant women tested had Bt toxin from GMO corn in their blood. (This corn was genetically engineered to produce Bt toxin in order to be insect resistant.) Sadly, so did 80 percent of their unborn fetuses. What is reassuring is that GMO labeling and non-GMO labeling is becoming more common in the United States and European Union, increasing transparency for the consumer. In the United States, you can look for either a "Non GMO Project Verified" label or a USDA Organic label to let you know your food is free of GMOs.

The Art of Processing Foods

Processing food goes back thousands of years. Foods such as ghee, butter, cheese, yoghurt, fermented foods, olive oil, and bread are a few examples of foods that have been naturally processed for millennia. More fundamentally, cooking is easily the most common processing technique. Adding heat to food has the ability to alter the structure of proteins, fats, and carbohydrates in food.

Processing food is not an inherently bad thing. If done wisely, this can improve the compatibility and digestibility of a food. If done incorrectly, it can produce a number of harmful byproducts.

One of the simplest natural processing methods includes soaking or sprouting beans, legumes, grains, nuts, and seeds to remove some of the more inflammatory compounds like lectins and make them easier to digest. Remember how the diets of all the longevity cultures I visited are extremely high in lectin-rich foods? Their traditional preparations of those foods also naturally minimize the lectin content. Soaking and boiling removes nearly all the lectins in beans, for example. And by skinning tomatoes, removing the seeds, and boiling them, as is often practiced in Sardinia, nearly all lectins are removed. This is an example where processing through sufficient heat improves the nutritional value of food.

If we compare the processing methods employed by the elders 80 years ago with modern, commercial food processing in industrialized nations, we find dramatic differences. Cristina Castillo of Guanacaste asserted, "We didn't have unhealthy foods. You know why? Because there wasn't as much commercialization of food. There wasn't big business." It is clear that today, we have prioritized speed, profit, taste, and convenience over food quality and health. Many of the processes that have been invented or highly utilized over the past hundred years are significantly altering the information contained within food in a way that does not serve human health.

Unnecessary sterilization of food and high use of pesticides have severely limited the microbial diversity of food, which ultimately hinders microbial communication from the environment to our microbiota. In addition, ultra-high pressure and heat have the ability to alter the protein, carbohydrate, and fat complexes in ways that research has shown to be very problematic. For example, with too much heat and pressurization, fats and oils can become oxidized, wreaking havoc on the body at the cellular level. Common toxic byproducts that occur with modern food processing include the following:

- *Acrylamide* is formed when asparagine, an amino acid in some foods, reacts with sugars at high temperatures. Research has repeatedly shown the ill effects of acrylamide, and the World Health Organization warned that it may be responsible for up to one third of all cancers caused by diet. Some acrylamide-heavy foods include French fries, some commercial cereals, potato chips, cookies, and crackers.

- *Heterocyclic amines*, which are carcinogenic, form when meats are heated at high temperatures for extended periods of time.

- *Nitrosamines* are formed when processed meats preserved with sodium nitrite are heated, as the sodium nitrite combines with proteins to form this toxic byproduct.

The other major challenges that have arisen over the last half century involve the preserving and packaging of food. There are so many preservatives, additives, artificial colors, artificial sweeteners, and extracts that it becomes overwhelming to think about. While governmental agencies consider these additives safe, there is plenty of research demonstrating the harmful effects of many of these non-food ingredients. And if you consider the combinatory and cumulative effect of consuming potentially hundreds of these ingredients daily, over the course of months or years, it's anybody's guess what the total health burden might look like.

There is a very long list of issues created by modern processing and preservation methods, and they all directly change the information contained within food to which your body responds. If foods are cooked, pressurized, sterilized, or altered in any way, there is a chance of creating damaging byproducts. Just about all these ingredients and byproducts will disrupt your gut microbiota, impair gut integrity, and decrease immune tolerance, which ultimately increases systemic inflammation and the likelihood of developing food sensitivities.

In general, our goal here is to incorporate minimally processed, organic, non-GMO whole foods in your diet as much as possible. Quality is key. Avoid or minimize packaged food all together. When you do opt for the packaged food, it's best to go organic and avoid any products with unfamiliar additives and ingredients. The more you can source food directly from your environment, just as the elders did for most of their lives, the better off you're likely to be.

THE TROUBLE WITH GRAINS

There are countless books published in the United States alone on the issues posed by gluten, wheat, and grains in general. Many people have clear physical symptoms from eating gluten, wheat, and other grains. In fact, I used to be one of them. There is an undeniable issue with grains and grain-based products in the industrialized countries around the world. In Okinawa and Guanacaste, cereal grains were only occasionally consumed. And for what it's worth, none of the elders had heard of anybody with sensitivities to any foods when they were young, including grains. According to the elders in Ikaria, grains and bread also posed no health issues for them over the past 100 years, as bread was commonly consumed. But none of the other cultures ate as much bread as the Sardinians.

It was fascinating to hear the Sardinians talk about bread and how important it was to them. There was no amount of research I could show them to convince them bread could in any way be harmful. The past 100 years of their own life experiences suggested otherwise. They did firmly acknowledge that the source grains and breadmaking processes had changed, however. Dr. Giovanni Ugas of Sardinia recalled the old way of making bread. He said, "Wheat was of high quality, so it was much tastier. It was produced in each family. That is, it was milled in the house. Women would get up early before dawn, at three or four in the morning. All of the processes were different than today. The taste of the wheat and the flour was different. Wheat was milled with the use of a donkey in the house, itself, until the 1950s and '60s. It was a local production, homemade. So it was a much, much tastier bread. Many things changed after the '50s. All of the production—so many of the vegetables that were produced until the '50s, changed."

If grains and bread inherently have always posed such an egregious threat to human health, it's hard to imagine why they would be so abundantly used in almost every culture around the world for thousands of years. Even in the United States, the epicenter of the gluten-free movement, wheat and gluten were only identified as problematic maybe 65 years ago or so. And in the past 20 years, issues with gluten have exploded to unprecedented levels. It seems there is more to the story. There are four primary issues with wheat in the modern world:

- First, large-scale use of pesticides like Roundup on wheat and other crops destroys gut microbiota, hampers digestion, and creates leaky gut.

- Second, most of the wheat flours that are used in commercial goods are highly refined white flours, not the entire grain.

- Third, modern grains usually aren't soaked or sprouted before being ground.

- Fourth, modern semidwarf wheat species are novel and created in a lab. They have been genetically modified to create high yields and resist pesticides, resulting in a crop that is quite different than the ancient grains used in Sardinia.

Many people continue to face health challenges with grains, even when they switch to organic wheat. One reason is that the body has been systemically assaulted for years by pesticide-laden, genetically modified wheat products, causing a damaged gut and an inability to digest gluten. The other major culprit is a result of gastrointestinal infections. It is possible to overcome gluten sensitivity over time by clearing potential infections, improving the integrity of the gut, improving your immune tolerance, and switching to more ancient species of wheat and grain. Until then, if grains are causing you issues, it is best to avoid grains until optimal gut and immune function is restored.

OPTIMIZING YOUR DIET

As you head for the produce aisle of a grocery store in the United States, the array of fresh produce is astounding. No matter what time of year, you can find upward of 50 or 60 common fruits and vegetables. Thanks to an amazing food distribution system, most people have access to foods grown from all over the world. While this is quite a luxury to have, it makes it that much more difficult to determine what one ideally *should* eat to maintain health. With the variety of dietary advice that can be found in books and on the Internet, it can be very difficult for the average person to discern what to believe. Tremendous guidance can certainly be found, but there is only one person who knows the answer—you. There may be foods that you used to be able to eat without issue that are now causing you problems. Or they may be medicine for your friend, but problematic for you.

The appropriate foods for you depend on your individual context—your age, health status, unique constitution, time of day, geography, season, objective, and lifestyle. Your body will speak to you if you practice tuning in and really pay attention to the language of the body. Pregnant women are wonderful case study examples. A woman's senses and intuition can be extremely heightened during pregnancy. Without knowing why, they will often crave certain foods they don't normally eat and detest other foods they normally have no problem with.

For the rest of us, there are many things to observe in our daily life to help give us clues:

- How does your mood change with different foods?

- Do you feel achy anywhere on your body?

- How is your sleep affected?

- How are your energy levels and cognitive function at different times of the day?

- Do you get constipated, bloated, or gassy? If so, when?

- Look to your skin for clues. When do you break out, feel itchy or dry, or otherwise have complaints?

Rely on your intuition—your inner knowing—for guidance. Trust it. Your body is communicating to you all the time. I invite you to get curious. Bring awareness to the subtle or not-so-subtle messages the body is sending, then take an honest assessment and adjust. This is a never-ending process because your context is always changing over time.

CONSIDER AYURVEDIC PRINCIPLES

There are many valid, modern dietary frameworks that exist and can be helpful for certain people in certain contexts. Yet I have found only one dietary framework sophisticated enough to work for everyone: Ayurveda. One of the beautiful things about Ayurveda is that its principles can be used to support any other modern dietary framework as well, including vegetarian, vegan, paleo, ketogenic, Atkins, macrobiotic, and Whole30. No matter what your dietary philosophy is, Ayurveda can help tailor it to you.

The dietary principles taught in Ayurveda have been around for thousands of years and are used all over the planet. They are individualized based primarily on your individual constitution and the existing imbalances you are currently experiencing. The framework also takes into consideration circadian rhythm and factors in seasonal changes. Ayurveda is a vast science that has mapped out many health concepts that modern science has only understood in the past 100 years!

While a deep dive into Ayurveda is beyond the scope of this book, I encourage you to take the first step to learn your constitution. The most accurate method is finding a good practitioner who can read your pulse to determine your constitution and identify your imbalances. You can also find questionnaires online that can help you determine your constitution, although they are not as accurate as an Ayurvedic practitioner. The Ayurvedic Institute created a short and easy questionnaire to get you started, which can be found at ayurveda.com.

Once you know your constitution, you can begin eating foods that help to balance out your natural dominant traits. The science of Ayurveda has mapped out how each food impacts each one of the three dominant traits or "doshas," known as vata, pitta, and kapha. You can find a food chart at ayurveda.com to help you remember which foods are more optimal for you.

What most people find in this exploration of Ayurveda is that some of their favorite and most frequently eaten foods are working to create greater imbalance—no matter how "healthy" the food is thought to be. When I learned that my favorite food and beverages like coffee, garlic, spinach, chia seeds, eggs, salsa, macadamia nuts, and dark chocolate were all exaggerating my dominant trait and increasing systemic imbalance, it made so much sense why I couldn't fully resolve my symptoms. Then I learned that foods like avocado, blueberries, asparagus, cilantro, basil, fennel, sweet potatoes, and ghee, among others, essentially acted as medicine for me, helping to bring my entire system back into balance.

When you finally have a complete map to work with, diet becomes so much simpler to navigate given your unique context, conditions, and objectives.

DIVERSITY AND THE MICROBIOME

Food is one of the most critical and consistent signals that inform our gut ecosystem about our local environment. But if the microbiota population in your GI tract is constantly under assault from disharmonious lifestyle and food choices, imbalance can take hold in the gut and the communication inevitably breaks down. In order to benefit from the energetic information and value of food, we must have a gut ecosystem that can decipher the information and translate it to our mitochondria and human DNA for healthy and harmonious genetic expression.

There is a large body of research that continues to demonstrate that greater diversity of microbial species in your GI tract translates to better health outcomes across the board. Studies show that gut microbiota diversity is low in nearly all chronic conditions. While all the precise mechanisms and associations haven't been fully worked out, there is a big effort to study individual species of microbes to see how they influence gut function and overall health.

The bottom line is that improving diversity is a worthwhile endeavor and will ultimately provide greater flexibility and a more robust capacity to deal with changing environmental conditions. Whether the elders knew it or not, each of their lifestyles and cultural cuisines were highly effective at increasing microbiota diversity and harmony with the local environment, allowing for balanced epigenetic expression and greater biological coherence.

Follow the Seasons

One of the most surefire ways to harmonize with the rhythms of nature, increase diversity in your diet, and increase gut microbiota diversity is to let your local seasons guide you. When visiting a preschool of three-, four-, and five-year-olds in Okinawa, I noticed a chart that was used to teach the kids which foods grew in each season. It surprised me to find that this was something they found important enough to teach preschoolers. When I asked the teacher about it, she said it was a very important part of their culture because it teaches them not only which foods grow in season, but the larger concepts that seasons represent. Rather than focusing on any specific group of foods as being notably healthier than others, they follow nature to determine which foods are more advantageous in a given season. The science of Ayurveda speaks of foods that grow in spring balancing out foods harvested in fall/winter; foods that are harvested in summer/fall balance out foods harvested in spring. Thus, the body is naturally kept in balance year after year.

As it were, the global food distribution network allows a New Yorker to eat bananas and broccoli in winter or fresh cucumbers in spring. But if you removed the idea of refrigeration and global shipping of food, nature's seasons would force us to eat seasonally. While this might seem to restrict foods in the diet, what you find is the exact opposite. Most people in Western industrial societies only eat a handful of whole foods and we tend to eat the same foods year-round in habitual form. But the elders were much more connected to their food and the seasons in which they grew. They had staples that they were able to consume all year, but the fruits, tubers, herbs, and vegetables rotated throughout the year in alignment with nature. This may seem like a minor detail to most, but this divergence from nature's cycles has repercussions that make a big difference to your health over time. Scientific research, the elders, and Ayurveda all agree—eating with the seasons is a wise thing to do.

According to scientific records, our ancient ancestors ate almost everything you can imagine, and many cultures around the world still do. Depending on the region and season, diets would include tuberous roots, fungi, fruit, vegetables, insects, sea creatures, birds, and land mammals of all kinds. Humans have a remarkable ability to adapt and thrive in just about any environment. If we weren't able to digest it, we found clever ways to predigest or prepare the food so we could digest it. Our ancestors would grind, ferment, soak, sprout, cook, and combine ingredients in an effort to preserve and maximize the availability of nourishment that their local environment provided. It's estimated that a hunter-gatherer population would typically consume upward of 600 different foods annually. Conversely, people in the United States today consume only 15 to 30 different foods on average.

While food diversity is not an absolute requirement for health, research has continued to show that as we reduce variety in our diet, we tend to see poor microbial diversity in our gastrointestinal tract. Poor diversity can reduce your ability to extract nutrients from food, increase the likelihood of microbial imbalance, reduce our ability to functionally adapt to a changing environment, and often results in immune dysregulation. Remember, the microbes you host in your gut will influence mitochondrial function, gene expression, neurotransmitter production, inflammation control, hormone balance, detoxification, and just about every cellular function imaginable. In this way, consuming a wide variety of foods in your diet will undoubtedly serve you well.

If your GI tract doesn't house the correct microbes or they aren't able to express a specific set of genetic codes, you may not be able to take full advantage of the benefits of a given food, no matter how healthy it is thought to be. By interacting with your local environment and food-based microorganisms by eating with the seasons, you better harmonize with nature to make best use of the food that grows around you.

Chapter 6

DIGESTION AND ELIMINATION

One who maintains a balanced state of the main elements
of the body, adequate digestion, proper excretion, blissful
condition of the soul, satisfied senses, and a happy state
of mind is called a healthy person.

— Vedic Sushruta sutra, Chapter 15, verse 41

Is there a concept in health and longevity more fundamental, more preeminent than digestion? Be it thought, emotion, food, or any other experience, adequate digestion is required for sustained health and well-being. When digestion is suboptimal, disease is sure to follow.

The process of effective digestion involves the intake of one substance and transforming it into a completely different substance. The mechanisms required to transfer the life-force energy from a plant into the life-force energy of a human is nothing short of magic. Western science has identified a handful of the biochemical reactions involved, most notably the citric acid cycle and mitochondrial respiration, for which a number of Nobel Prizes have been awarded over the past 70 years. While the tremendous knowledge we've gained of these processes is proving to be very important, we still don't fully understand the immense complexity involved.

It is easy to take the process of digestion for granted. After all, we eat food every day and eventually excrete the waste, all without giving it much thought. Yet digestive disorders are one of the most common ailments in the United States, affecting 60 million to 70 million adults, according to research from 2018. Surveys indicate that upward of 74 percent of Americans are living with gastrointestinal discomfort.

Over the past 20 years in particular, the microbiome has become hot topic in natural health circles and in mainstream academic research. The scientific studies continue to focus heavily on the deep biochemistry involved with microbiota, secondary metabolites, gut-brain connections, the gut-immune axis, probiotics, prebiotics, and the like. This has been fantastically useful for the development of new pharmaceuticals, patented probiotics, targeted supplements, medical procedures, and the use of specific plant extracts to benefit gastrointestinal health. With respect to the latter, it is interesting to note that modern scientific research is frequently confirming the specific benefits and uses of a variety of herbs used in Ayurvedic, Chinese, and indigenous medicine for hundreds or even thousands of years. There is far less incentive, however, to invest in scientific research that examines the role of lifestyle factors and dietary habits that affect digestion. For this, Ayurveda carries a lot of wisdom, as optimizing digestion is a core principle of maintaining health in the Vedic texts.

The subsequent side of the digestive story is elimination. Even if digestion is optimized, we must maintain effective and thorough elimination of all the wastes that are naturally produced as a result of digestion of food, daily living, and cellular metabolic activity. But as is the case for nearly everyone, there will be times, perhaps frequently, that digestion and efficient metabolic activity remains suboptimal or downright poor. In these circumstances, optimizing elimination becomes even more imperative to avoid the rapid accumulation of toxic wastes throughout the body.

A simple analogy might be to think of your home environment. Each one of us produces a certain amount of trash as a result of our normal daily living. Some households produce a lot of trash, while others produce less, depending on a number of factors. In order to keep your house clean, it can be helpful to focus your efforts on producing less trash and frequently tidying. However, if you don't take out the trash, or you do so at a slower rate than you produce it, eventually the accumulated mess will occupy your house in ways that become meaningfully disruptive and prevent you from carrying out normal daily activities. An odor is likely to develop. Bacteria, mold, and other organisms may show visible signs of growth and accumulation in an attempt to decompose organic matter. A similar concept applies to your biological systems. While your body contains natural intelligence and mechanisms to eliminate waste that accumulates in the GI tract, inside your cells, and throughout the body, these systems can become impaired and bogged down over time. And for many, there is a tremendous opportunity to dramatically improve health by taking an active role in optimizing both digestion and elimination in the gastrointestinal tract, at the cellular level, and even with respect to thoughts and emotions.

OPTIMIZING YOUR DIGESTION

The phrase "you are what you eat" should probably be replaced with "you are what you digest"! When you harmonize your diet and lifestyle choice in ways that don't overburden and extinguish your body's digestive capacity—or perhaps even learn to enhance it—health is your reward. When digestion is impaired, the very act of eating food, which should nourish and help build life, may instead be causing disease and contributing to your own demise. In Ayurveda, it is said that impaired or imbalanced *agni* (which can be thought of as digestion, metabolization, and intelligence) is at the core of all disease. And when *agni* is extinguished, death is sure to follow.

There are a few factors that inhibit digestion of food:

- Eating when thirsty, bored, or emotionally disturbed.
- Eating large meals first thing in the morning or late at night, when digestion is weak.

- Consuming cold drinks during meals or in between meals.

- Vigorous exercise less than an hour before a meal, during a meal, or within 90 minutes of finishing a meal.

- Eating quickly without chewing your food thoroughly.

- Eating to excess.

Fortunately, there are a great number of things you can do to optimize digestion:

- Eat only when truly hungry.

- Choose organic, whole foods and prepare them properly.

- See and smell your food before eating.

- Eat with loved ones.

- Eat slowly and with intention.

- Eat on a regular schedule.

The first component of digestion is having hunger already present in the body before you eat. This may sound obvious, but true hunger is a key signal that the body is ready for a meal. With hunger usually comes a greater secretion of saliva, optimal levels of hydrochloric acid in the stomach, increased production of digestive enzymes, bile, pancreatic fluids, and ability to absorb and assimilate your meal. If you're snacking all the time, your body isn't capable of thoroughly digesting the food you're eating, leading to increased inflammation in the GI tract and eventually throughout the whole body.

The second component of good digestion is to choose organic, whole foods and prepare them properly as was discussed in the previous chapter. Highly processed foods tend to lose their biological complexity and natural intelligence that comes in the form of enzymes, microbes, and beneficial phytochemicals with which the human digestive system has coevolved and often benefits from. And foods that contain man-made chemicals and artificial ingredients have the capacity to disrupt gut microbiota and mitochondria, create gastrointestinal inflammation, and excessively tax organs of elimination.

The third component involves the precephalic phase of digestion. When you are hungry and preparing food, the digestive process is sufficiently enhanced as you see, smell, or even think about your food. If you've ever walked into a restaurant or home and noticed your mouth watering from the rich fragrance of your favorite meal, you know what I mean. This is the precephalic phase of digestion in action. It is ideal to regularly prepare and cook meals at home, which helps to activate digestive function for anybody that can see or smell the food before it hits their plate.

The fourth and fifth component center around the social aspect of food. In this regard, there are two somewhat opposing ways to enhance digestion. One way is to eat among friends or family in a cordial or festive way that involves lots of chatter, laughing, music, and good spirit. The jovial nature helps to relax the sympathetic nervous system and activate the parasympathetic (rest and digest) nervous system. And because of the conversational activity, most people tend to eat more slowly. This was common among the elders around the world, particularly in Ikaria and Sardinia, and to a lesser degree in Costa Rica.

The fifth component depends on focusing your awareness on the act of eating—chewing, tasting, and digesting. We noticed that the Okinawan culture adopted a bit more of this style of eating practice, though not exclusively. Where your awareness goes, energy and blood flows. And where you send blood, you send function. Bringing awareness to the entire aspect of eating will consciously assist the largely unconscious process of digestion. Taste receptors on the tongue are not merely for entertainment. They serve critical roles in signaling to the body what kind of food is on its way and what will be needed to digest it. By consciously connecting to these taste sensations, you can enhance the communication signals sent to the brain and the rest of the body.

There is a useful adage to remember when it comes to chewing your food, "chew your liquids and drink your solids." When you mindfully and thoroughly chew your food, not only will you better break down food from the mechanical perspective, but you will better coat your food with saliva, thereby increasing the enzymatic breakdown. The enzymes found in saliva are not a trivial part of the process. One such salivary enzyme is DPP-IV, which has been scientifically shown to break down gluten, among other food proteins.

Regardless of the social setting, your meals are an opportunity to slow down the mind. It is the perfect time to take a break from the fast-paced environments and overstimulation that often accompanies work and other daily activities. It can even be helpful to say a little prayer, take a moment of gratitude, practice a short meditation, or do some breathing exercises, such as the 4-7-8 breath, to help transition from your typical daily activities to eating your meal. This will help activate the parasympathetic (rest and digest) nervous system and calm the sympathetic nervous system. By bringing as much conscious awareness to the entire process of eating, bite by bite, you can enhance digestion and assimilation significantly. Research also shows this helps you better recognize when you are satiated, reducing the likelihood of overeating.

The sixth primary component of good digestion is related to circadian rhythm. Recall from Chapter 4 that your body is trying to predict the future based on a series of entrainment cues that include light, temperature, exercise, and food. We are highly adaptive creatures and the more consistency you can provide with respect to the timing of these stimuli, the better your body can anticipate function.

Regularly scheduling your meals can feel a bit antithetical to the idea of only eating when you are hungry. However, if you find yourself hungry before your next meal, scheduling your meals and optimizing circadian rhythm can slowly influence the hormones and metabolic functions that trigger hunger, so they begin to align with your scheduled mealtimes. If you find that you're not hungry when it comes time for a meal, such as lunch, you can consider reducing the size of your breakfast the following day or skipping breakfast all together. Indeed, the timing of your meals is so important, it has its own guidelines.

Eat On Time

While most of the attention in the health world is focused on *what* you should eat, there is a lot to gain when you really learn *when* you should eat. Generally speaking, the advice of current scientific literature, Ayurvedic science, and the wisdom of the elders agree on these fundamental rules:

- Eat two to three main meals, roughly between the hours of 6 A.M. and 6 P.M.

- Fast for at least 12 hours overnight.

- Eat your largest meal of the day at lunch or an early dinner.

- Wait at least 90 minutes after your meal to engage in heavy physical exertion or evening sleep.

These are rather simple concepts on paper, yet they can be difficult to implement in a busy modern society that involves a 9-to-5 job, happy hours, dinners out, birthday parties, vending machines, air travel, concerts, and sporting events. While perfection is not required, consistently following these guidelines can make a huge difference in your health over the long-term.

Fasting may sound like an intimidating undertaking, but remember this number of hours includes your sleeping period, when you are naturally not eating. Then, while you are awake, you may drink water or tea without breaking your fast. According to research, consistent 12- to 18-hour fasting periods and short periods of significant caloric restriction can lead to better mitochondrial function, improved microbiota diversity in the gut, effective blood sugar control, improved cellular detoxification, and greater cellular repair. It is important to give your digestive system a break from food and alcohol so it can do its own cleaning and repair. Digestion is a lot of work, and when you give your body a break, it can dedicate more energy to other systems of the body.

For those who are hypoglycemic or diabetic (type 1), it can certainly be helpful to snack a few times throughout the day to maintain blood sugar regularity. But for most of the population, eating two or three meals a day is best, ideally eating only when truly hungry. Many individuals find that hunger doesn't show up until late morning or lunch. If this is the case, you can skip breakfast, thereby prolonging your fasting period. For those who eat breakfast and a large lunch, then go to bed early, skipping dinner could be a good option. It is important to also keep in mind that thirst can show up as a false hunger signal, particularly in the morning. Presumed hunger pangs may disappear after drinking some water.

Returning to the idea of circadian biology and the natural cyclical function of your body, digestive capacity also follows this rhythm. If you're synchronized with the solar cycle, your digestive fire will burn the hottest near the hottest part of the day. The solar fire and your digestive fire are yoked. With this in mind, it is wise to have your largest meal between roughly 11 A.M. and 3 P.M. for optimal digestion. In the morning and evening, when digestion is weaker, opt for smaller meals so as not to overburden your reduced digestive capacity.

Eat in Moderation

There is a famous Tibetan proverb that says, "Eat half, walk double, laugh triple, and love without measure." From my experience of the elders, I think they would wholeheartedly agree with this sentiment. Ikarian local George Stenos, who at the age of 92 was as sharp and lively as anybody 30 years his junior, told me, "First of all, I don't eat much. I eat my meal on a small plate. I don't eat much meat. I follow the Mediterranean diet, and in general, a healthy lifestyle." In Okinawa, they have a dedicated phrase to communicate the idea of how much food should be eaten: *hara hachi bu*. This is the practice of eating until you are 80 percent full.

There was another aspect to the elders' way of eating that I noticed when examining the historical context of their life. Because they had to work to grow, harvest, raise, or hunt their food, there was a direct relationship between the work they did and the food they consumed. This sets up a self-regulating mechanism that prevents overproduction and overconsumption of food. There is a disincentive to consistently overeat because they would then only have to work harder to produce more food. As such, the elders generally got by on what they needed to be healthy and satisfied while also recognizing the health benefits of eating in moderation.

Ayurvedic wisdom also has a guiding principle that conveys this principle. It is said that you should stop eating when your stomach is $1/3$ full of food, $1/3$ full of liquid, $1/3$ full of air. While it is impossible to follow this advice literally, the concept helps to communicate and regulate a few aspects of eating.

- First, you shouldn't overeat because that will overwhelm your digestive fire (*agni*) and cause you to improperly digest your food. Roughly two handfuls of food is a good rule of thumb.

- Second, do not drink too much liquid during your meal, as it hinders digestion. Sipping a little warm water or ginger tea, on the other hand, can actually improve digestion. However, even from a Western scientific perspective, it is acknowledged that ingesting too much liquid will dilute stomach acid, resulting in a more alkaline stomach environment that is not ideal for digestion.

- And the final idea of Ayurveda's rule of thirds is that you want to leave some space in your stomach to allow for the proper mixing and metabolic activity within the stomach. By slowly eating your meal, you'll be better at gauging how full you are so you can stop short of overeating.

Once again, we see that the elders, modern science, and Ayurvedic wisdom are all in alignment with regard to digestion.

Aid Digestion with Ayurvedic Herbs

There are three main spices used in Ayurveda to support digestion in a balanced way for everybody. You can combine the seeds of cumin, coriander, and fennel (CCF) in equal parts and make a tea. Regularly drinking a little of this CCF before a meal, after a meal, or in between meals can be very effective at improving digestion as well as a number of gastrointestinal symptoms and conditions.

Black pepper and turmeric work well together to improve digestion as they have a combinatory effect. Black pepper has been shown to stimulate digestion, and turmeric helps to reduce gastrointestinal inflammation.

Raw ginger is one of the more powerful digestive foods, activating the migrating motor complex in the small intestine, which helps to move food matter through the GI tract by facilitating good gastric motility and gastric emptying. You can make ginger tea and sip before, during, after, and between meals. You can also make a little pickled ginger by peeling and slicing a few pieces of ginger and soaking it in a brine of lime juice and a few pinches of salt. Keep this in the fridge and have a small slice before and after meals.

There are a number of other herbs and spices that can be beneficial for different aspects of digestion, assimilation, and overall GI health. Anise seed, peppermint leaf, artichoke, dill, gentian, cardamom, caraway, lemon balm, cinnamon, slippery elm, marshmallow root, and calendula are commonly used in herbal medicine to improve digestion and gastrointestinal health. You may find it helpful to add some of these herbs to your meal or drink tea throughout the day using a variety of these herbs. Know your Ayurvedic constitution and follow an Ayurvedic food chart to select the best herbs for your unique context to avoid creating imbalance.

Quick Tips for Aiding Digestion

There are a number of other tricks to help activate and facilitate good digestion throughout the day and night.

Before you eat: Thirty minutes prior to a meal, drink a small cup of warm water and then go for a 10- to 15-minute walk. Not only will this help you determine if your hunger was really thirst, it will also hydrate your tissues and awaken the digestive process, improve blood and lymph circulation, and clear metabolic waste from the system in preparation for the hard work of digestion that is about to follow.

After you eat: Rest for 10 to 15 minutes after a meal. Lying on your left side will encourage optimal blood circulation, improve lymphatic flow, bile flow, support spleen function, and movement of food material into and through the colon.

If you tend to get tired after meals, instead of resting it may be best to go for a short walk. In addition to supporting digestion, this will also help to balance blood sugar and insulin levels.

When you sleep: Sleeping on your left side at night will also improve digestion. For those with gastrointestinal disorders, sleeping on your left side may have a noticeable effect if done regularly.

UNDERSTANDING YOUR BODY'S TOXIC LOAD

As a result of normal daily function, we all create a toxic, morbid waste product in our cells and various tissues throughout the body, including in the GI tract. Beyond our normal production of digestive and metabolic waste, it is not uncommon to have an elevated production of gastrointestinal and metabolic waste due to a variety of imbalances, such as: insufficient production of hydrochloric acid in the stomach, inadequate digestive enzymes, poor gastrointestinal motility, gut microbiota imbalances, emotional disturbances, mental stress, environmental chemicals and metals, infections, poor circadian rhythm, or anything else that might impair thorough digestion and efficient cellular metabolism. The more impaired your digestion and cellular metabolization is, the more toxic cellular waste is naturally produced.

Aside from the inherent digestive and metabolic wastes produced by our body, one can also face a high load of biotoxins produced by the organisms that live within us. Yeasts, molds, bacteria, and parasites of all kinds produce biotoxins that our bodies must deal with. Common biotoxins include mycotoxins, endotoxins such as lipopolysaccharides, and volatile organic compounds. These can build up in tissues throughout the body and place added burden on all organs of elimination.

Another major toxic load on the body comes from environmental exposure. Nobody knows how many chemicals are currently in use today around the planet. However, the Environmental Protection Agency has over 80,000 chemicals on record. And from biopsies, it currently estimated that the average Western human has somewhere between 20,000 and 30,000 chemicals stored in the body. To put things in context, surveys have been done by the Environmental Working Group suggesting that, on average, men use about 6 personal care products each day and women use around 12. Through the use of these common products, the average exposure is over 150 man-made chemicals each day. Finally, in a study of the cord blood from 10 babies born in 2004, researchers found an average of 200 industrial chemicals and pollutants. The three pollutants found in every baby included lead, mercury, and PCBs. Unlike in the 1930s and '40s, when the elders were kids living in remote areas of the planet, modern humans are facing an unprecedented exposure to heavy metals and man-made chemicals—much of which occurs through the skin and in our food, beverages, medications, and drinking water.

In a supremely healthy gastrointestinal tract, there is an intelligent and highly effective barrier that prevents foreign invaders and inflammatory agents from entering the blood stream. But when there is an accumulation of metabolic waste, infections, biotoxins, man-made chemicals, and metals in the gastrointestinal tract can often migrate from the safe confines of the GI tract throughout the body, settling in various tissues and negatively effecting cellular metabolic activity in these areas, which further impairs cellular intelligence, communication, and efficiency. The accumulation of waste products in various tissues throughout the body will eventually lead to any number of chronic diseases. In fact, in Ayurveda it is commonly said that *ama* (i.e., toxic metabolic waste) is the root cause of all disease. In this way, a large part of the work in Ayurvedic medicine is to clear accumulated toxic waste out of the system and to kindle a robust and balanced *agni* (i.e., digestion and metabolism).

There are similar ideas described by Western science as well. For example, it is widely demonstrated in the research that unmetabolized food proteins, toxic byproducts generated in the GI tract, infectious agents, and man-made chemicals can cause or contribute to a hyperpermeable, or "leaky," gut, resulting in a loss of barrier integrity and ushering in inflammatory agents and undigested food proteins into the blood stream. This often results in a complex orchestra of excessive inflammation and dysregulated immune function that can have catastrophic results over time. These inflammogens, or antigens that migrate from the GI tract into the blood stream, can then cause damage to various organs and tissues throughout the body and can also set the stage for immune cross-reactivity and eventually autoimmunity. This is just one simplified example of what may result from poorly digested food, from the Western scientific perspective. There are many other pathologies that may result as well, including gastrointestinal damage, small intestinal bacterial overgrowth, gastrointestinal infections, liver dysfunction, gall bladder stagnation, endocrine disruption, neuroinflammation, cardiovascular disease, metabolic syndromes, and many more.

Modern Western science also describes dysfunctional processes at the cellular level caused by an accumulation of chemicals, metals, metabolic waste, lack of sleep, poor circadian rhythm, mental-emotional stress, and the like. These factors lead to excessive oxidative stress, mitochondrial dysfunction, and damage to DNA, cell membranes, and other cellular architecture—all of which impair metabolic function and reduce cellular intelligence, just as Ayurveda describes.

Reduce Your Toxin Exposure

One of the most important aspects of supporting elimination is to reduce the load of inflammatory agents that make their way into the body. Unfortunately, these agents are nearly everywhere in the modern world—far too many to list here. However, you can see vast improvement in your health by focusing on the following:

- Filter your drinking water or source from a clean spring.
- Reduce your consumption of industrially processed foods of all kinds.
- Eat organic and wild-caught foods or grow your own.
- Consider having a skilled biological dentist remove any metal amalgams.
- Have a skilled biological dentist address any dental infections or oral imbalances.
- Reduce personal care products that contain industrial chemicals, especially cosmetics.
- Reduce your use of cleaning products that contain industrial chemicals.
- Address any potential mold exposure in the home or office.
- Eliminate or reduce any unnecessary pharmaceutical drugs.
- Stop drinking out of plastic containers.

There's a cumulative biological effect caused by the pervasive and toxic milieu found in the sources above. Chronic disease happens gradually, then suddenly. As the body's function declines and the compounding effect of hundreds of chemicals and metals persist, at some point the burden becomes too much for the body to effectively compensate. That's when crisis appears as if out of nowhere.

OPTIMIZING YOUR ELIMINATION PROCESSES

Both Ayurveda and modern Western science point to the general idea that an accumulation of unmetabolized waste products and inflammatory agents in the GI tract and at the cellular level will increase inflammation, impair cellular communication, and result in greater damage and disease. This is why digestion and elimination both in the GI tract and at the cellular level are such important parts of the health equation. While the production of toxic metabolic waste is inevitable, there are a number of steps you can take to aid your body in clearing it.

Defecation

You can learn a great deal about monitoring your stool. The GI tract is where a great deal of disease begins, so learning to read the signs of when something is amiss can be an effective way to prevent long-term complication.

The consistency, color, and buoyancy of your stool will naturally vary. Ideally, you would like to see stool that is light brown in color, floats, slightly oily, not sticking to the bowl, with minimal odor, and the consistency of a ripe banana. If this long list of criteria is rarely met, you're not alone. It is helpful to know what is ideal, however.

Healthy fecal elimination should occur once or twice daily for the average adult. Ideally, as part of your morning routine, you would have a bowel movement within the first 30 minutes of waking up. Again, it isn't uncommon for this not to happen, but drinking warm water or tea upon waking can help initiate a bowel movement.

One herbal remedy for improving bowel regularity and overall gut health is the Ayurvedic formula triphala. This herbal formula is generally well tolerated, and its beneficial effects tend to increase with regular use over the course of weeks, months, and even years. Triphala is one of the most revered formulations in Ayurveda for its ability to gently cleanse, balance, and tonify the GI tract, improve digestion, and support healthy elimination. About 30 minutes before bed, you can take two to three tablets with a small glass of warm water. Or you can steep ½ teaspoon to 1 teaspoon of triphala powder in a cup of boiling water for 10 minutes, then drink.

Another important component of healthy gastrointestinal elimination and bowel regularity is the consumption of dietary fiber. Fiber works by drawing fluids from the body into the GI tract, adding bulk to the stool, and sweeping out toxic metabolic waste from the GI tract. Scientific research has demonstrated a wide range of benefits of both soluble and insoluble fiber that include tonifying the colon walls, improved absorption of nutrients, binding of toxic chemicals, improved blood sugar control, balancing cholesterol and triglyceride levels, and improved cardiovascular health. The long-term protective effects of regularly consuming sufficient levels of fiber are difficult to overstate.

The most effective and healthy long-term solution to get sufficient dietary fiber is not to consume fiber supplements but to regularly consume a wide variety of whole fruits and vegetables along with properly prepared beans, legumes, nuts, and seeds. The recommended daily intake of fiber tends to range around 25 grams for women and 35 grams for men. However, every individual must find their own unique balance and optimal amount of daily dietary fiber. Because insoluble fiber absorbs water and draws fluids into the GI tract, you may want to increase your water consumption between meals when increasing your intake of dietary fiber. The most effective gauge is to let your stool analysis and natural thirst guide you.

Hydration and Urination

It is difficult to overstate the role that your liver and kidneys play in maintaining effective elimination. It is estimated that the liver is responsible for over 500 vital functions and that the kidneys process over 50 gallons of fluid every day. The liver is responsible for breaking down, transforming, and removing chemicals, food additives, excess hormones, medications, and the like. The kidneys work to filter and excrete toxic waste that accumulates in the blood. As such, any effective detoxification or cleansing protocol will place a heavy burden on the liver and kidneys. Because of this, adequate daily hydration becomes critical as it lessens the burden on the liver and kidneys in their effort to biotransform and excrete toxins that can accumulate in the body and eventually find their way into the blood. Simply put, the solution to pollution is dilution.

The most effective way to stay hydrated without impairing digestion is to consistently sip warm water throughout the day. Warm rather than cold water is extremely beneficial because it requires no bodily energy to heat up before it is assimilated. Do not drink large amounts of water at once, as this has a negative effect on digestion, even away from meals. However, after you wake up in the morning and have cleaned your mouth, you can drink a larger amount of warm water, 16 to 24 ounces at once. Adding lemon or lime juice to your morning water also improves digestion and detoxification, particularly with respect to the liver and gall bladder.

Your urine color and clarity is also worth monitoring. In the morning, you will likely notice that it is a bit cloudier and darker colored than it should be during the day. If your urine is a dark yellow or orange during the day, it generally indicates you would benefit from drinking more water. On the flip side, if your urine is clear all the time, you are drinking too much water and may be excessively dumping minerals. Your urine color will naturally fluctuate, but generally it should be a mild to dark yellow and not particularly cloudy.

Sweating

The skin is the largest organ in the body, and it is anything but passive. Skin biology is quite complex and responsible for a great deal of function that is required for you to remain healthy. One of these very important functions is to excrete waste products through the process of sweating. You might even hear the skin referred to as your "third kidney," as perspiration assists the kidneys and liver in the elimination of a great deal of accumulated toxins.

Sweating on a regular basis helps to open your pores, increase exfoliation, revitalize the skin, and balance the skin's microbial population by eliminating chemicals, metals, and biotoxins from the body and dermal layers. In Ayurveda, it is said that sweating loosens waste from the deep tissues, improves circulation, and helps to move waste into the digestive tract for elimination, particularly when oil is applied to the skin prior to a good sweat.

A large body of research shows that sauna therapy mobilizes fat-stored toxins and increases excretion of arsenic, cadmium, lead, mercury, PCBs, dioxins, benzene, chlorinated pesticides, and a variety of other toxic substances. Research has also demonstrated that detoxification through sweating in a sauna can even exceed the amount of toxins filtered through the kidneys. It should be noted that bathing in a sauna has also been shown to improve cardiovascular health, boost growth hormone, reduce pain, improve insulin sensitivity, boost immune function, lower stress levels, and improve mood.

To maintain optimal health, it is beneficial for most people to have a 10- to 20-minute whole-body sweat at least once or twice a week. You can achieve this through exercise, dry sauna, infrared sauna, or steam bath. For those with an increased load of chemicals and metals or who may have poor excretion through the kidneys, achieving a full-body sweat on a regular basis can make a world of difference to their health.

Lymphatic Flow

The lymphatic system is often one of the most underappreciated and underrecognized systems of the body. This vast network of lymphatic tissues consists of fluid, vessels, ducts, fascia, nodes, and organs such as the spleen, appendix, bone marrow, thymus, tonsils, and adenoids. This network also involves critical components such as the gut-associated lymphoid tissue (GALT) in the gastrointestinal tract as well as the glymphatic tissue in the brain.

The fluids in your lymphatic system do not flow like blood in the cardiovascular system. Rather, they require bodily movement and exogenous pressure to effectively move, circulate, and eventually drain. One of the primary roles of your lymphatic system is to reclaim excess fluids that have drained from cells and tissues throughout the body and return them from the interstitium (fluid, fascia, and spaces between organs) to the blood stream.

Your lymphatic system is also an important part of your immune system, producing a variety of immune factors, trapping pathogens, and reducing the threat of infection. It also plays a critical role in dietary fat delivery and absorption. As such, maintaining healthy lymphatic flow is a critical aspect of elimination and clearing the body of accumulated waste products and damaged cells. When lymphatic flow and drainage becomes impaired, there is a greater risk of infectious disease as well as an increased body burden of toxic chemicals, metals, and biological waste products. Over time, poor lymphatic flow and drainage can contribute or directly lead to any number of chronic illnesses including chronic skin conditions, autoimmune conditions, joint issues, neurodegenerative diseases, chronic fatigue, and cancer.

The severity of lymph congestion can be quite difficult for one to gauge. Furthermore, determining the level of contribution that lymph stagnation may have on symptomology is also quite challenging. However, any improvement in lymphatic flow will invariably assist in your body's ability to return to a healthy, harmonious, and coherent state. Fortunately, there are simple things you can do to improve the health of your lymphatic tissue:

— *Maintain Adequate Hydration:* While lymph is composed of about 95 percent water, its composition is in constant flux as it exchanges contents between the blood and bodily tissues. Drinking warm water throughout the day and minimizing diuretics like caffeine and alcohol are foundational in maintaining good lymphatic flow.

— *Regular Movement:* Consistent movement and exercise may be one of the most important aspects of maintaining good health into old age. Not only does exercise stimulate sweating and increase blood flow, it also improves lymphatic drainage and increases respiration, both of which provide substantial assistance to the processes of detoxification and the flushing of metabolic waste. While rebounding or jumping has been shown to be highly effective for lymphatic drainage in particular, activities such as yoga, brisk walking, Pilates, qigong, resistance training, swimming, and many other forms of movement are beneficial as well.

— *Massage:* All forms of massage can be highly effective at manually moving lymph throughout the body. The body contains upward of 500 lymph nodes, and focusing on areas where they are clustered is particularly beneficial. These areas include the upper groin, armpits, sides of the neck, abdomen, and upper chest. Ideally, use strokes that move toward the heart.

— *Contrast Showers:* Another effective method of increasing both blood and lymph circulation is a hot and cold contrasting shower. In hot water, your blood vessels become dilated, allowing for greater flow to the peripheral tissues. Cold water has the opposite effect, causing blood flow to constrict to the peripheral tissues and shunt to your core. The sudden change in temperature when alternating between hot then cold water works to effectively contract and squeeze lymph throughout the body.

Cycle two or three times between cold and hot, maintaining at least a minute at each temperature. Try to take a contrast shower at least weekly.

There are a few contraindications when it comes to the use of alternating hot and cold showers, however. They should be avoided by those who are pregnant, who have a heart condition, or who have extreme adrenal dysregulation.

— *Dry Brushing:* Dry brushing is an ancient Ayurvedic technique that helps to exfoliate the skin, stimulate the lymphatic system, and increase blood circulation. Dry brushing a few times per week before your shower is preferred and typically involves the use of a silk glove to gently brush the skin, although any kind of natural cloth fiber can also be effective. Additionally, you can find a bristled brush specifically designed for dry brushing.

Start brushing at the feet or head, always brushing toward the heart. When brushing your legs, stroke toward the groin area. For the arms, brush toward your armpits. Use long, straight strokes on your limbs and circular strokes on your joints.

— *Deep Breathing:* As if there weren't enough reasons to focus on the breath, it can also be used to facilitate greater lymphatic flow. In particular, deep, diaphragmatic breathing into the belly through the nose helps to maintain parasympathetic tone while using your lungs and diaphragm to pull fluids from the primary lymph ducts into the blood stream with a vacuum effect. In fact, research has demonstrated that deep breathing pulls lymph up from the legs and is more effective than walking or jogging. When it comes to improving lymphatic flow, the most important aspect of the breath is a slow and silent full exhalation, drawing the belly in by forcing out the breath. Then, filling up the belly and lower rib cage without allowing the shoulders to raise. Several rounds of deep breathing each day can result in a huge improvement in lymphatic drainage.

Liver and Gall Bladder Support

A healthy and well-functioning liver and gall bladder are essential for proper digestion and metabolization of proteins, carbohydrates, and fats from food. They also play a critical role in eliminating toxic buildup in the tissues. One of the liver's main jobs is to enzymatically transform and neutralize toxic substances so they can be carried out of the body by the urine and bile produced by the gall bladder. If the liver is unable to successfully transform these toxins or the gallbladder is sluggish and can't produce sufficient bile, toxins will circulate in the blood stream and eventually get deposited in the liver, fat cells, bone marrow, joints, muscles, brain, and other tissues throughout the body.

One of the most effective ways to support the liver and gall bladder is through intermittent fasting. You'll be giving them a break from digesting foods on a regular basis if you fast 12 to 18 hours a day. Also consider short water or juice fasts of three to five days, if your health allows.

Common foods and herbs that support liver and gallbladder function include cruciferous vegetables, beets, carrots, apples, bitter greens, garlic, fenugreek, dandelion greens, cilantro, cucumber, artichoke, turmeric, fennel, cinnamon, and ginger.

There is a bile acid supplement on the market that is worth noting here as well. It is called tauroursodeoxycholic acid and is known as TUDCA. Its therapeutic use was influenced by the use of bear bile in traditional Chinese medicine. While the theory and use of bear bile in traditional Chinese medicine is quite different than the application of TUDCA today, researchers discovered in their analysis of bear bile that it contains a relatively high level of TUDCA and believe it is one of the reasons why bear bile was thought to be so effective in traditional Chinese medicine. And thus, as a substitute for harvesting and using bear bile, a synthetic form of TUDCA was developed—and it is proving to be highly effective in supporting healthy bile flow and improving the quality of bile. TUDCA has also been shown to protect mitochondria and support gut microbiota balance. While not a gallbladder cure-all, this bile acid derivative is quite safe for most adults and can provide substantial benefit for those with a sluggish liver and gallbladder.

Kidney Support

Nephrons are the functional tissues of the kidneys. And unlike liver tissue, when nephrons die, they cannot be regrown or repaired. Beyond filtering fluids, the kidneys also help regulate blood pressure, produce vitamin D, and balance electrolytes. So protecting the kidneys from assault and supporting kidney function is paramount. The most effective way to support the kidneys is to stay hydrated by drinking warm water throughout the day. Many of the foods that support the liver and gallbladder, listed previously, also support the kidneys. Other herbs include hydrangea root, gravel root, goldenrod, uva ursi, marshmallow root, parsley, and horsetail, among others.

FURTHER SUPPORT FOR DETOXIFICATION AND ELIMINATION

There are a great number of detoxification methods that involve actively pulling chemicals, metals, and pathogens out of the body tissues. When done under professional supervision, these methods can be fantastic for cleaning up the body. However, there is significant risk if done haphazardly and incorrectly. Always work with a skilled practitioner who has your confidence.

What should be first considered is the overall health state of the person. How much can the person handle and how well-functioning are their elimination pathways? It is critical to ensure the body is able to eliminate effectively before pulling toxins out of tissues and sending them into circulation. If there is stagnation within the GI tract, kidneys, skin, liver, gall bladder, and lymphatic system, it should be addressed first if possible before the active mobilization and transport of toxins.

Second, when it comes to mobilizing and transporting toxins out of tissues into circulation, it is always better to go too slow than too fast. Otherwise, for example, you may mobilize aluminum out of a relatively benign place in the body and have it end up getting transported to the brain, which is probably the worst place for it to end up. Or you may end up permanently damaging tissues like the kidneys if they are unable to keep up with excretion of metals. A tell-tale sign you're mobilizing toxins faster than you're eliminating them is when you experience a Jarisch-Herxheimer reaction, or detox reaction, which can involve any number of sudden symptoms ranging from skin inflammation to flu-like symptoms and worse. This is one of the reasons why various binding agents should be used in the process of eliminating chemicals, metals, and pathogens.

Third, there is always an order of operation that should be considered. In nearly all cases, toxic overload includes some combination of chemicals, metals, mold, or other parasitic infection. The combination and severity of these factors will determine which is addressed first before moving on to the next. These are just a few reasons to consider working with a skilled professional before attempting to pull toxins out of the deep tissues with concentrated and effective agents.

Binding Agents for Detoxification

Natural binding agents are one of the most effective ways of assisting the body's natural elimination pathways without introducing much risk. Because all modern humans (and animals, for that matter) are inherently exposed to a relatively high degree of man-made chemicals, heavy metals, and natural biological toxins, special consideration should be placed on regularly assisting the body's innate ability to escort toxins out of the body. When your body is working optimally, your intestinal tract, liver, gall bladder, and kidneys in particular are working in concert to transform, break down, and flush out toxins through the stool and urine.

However, there are many reasons why the body's natural detox function may become compromised. When this is the case, the overall toxic load can build up in the GI tract and throughout the body. Unfortunately, as the toxic load increases in your cells and tissues, detoxification function can become further compromised. This creates a vicious cycle of reduced function, increased toxic load, and more damage, followed by reduced function.

If detoxification function is normally good, a sudden increase in exposure of chemicals, metals, or biotoxins can quickly compromise your natural ability to detox well and kick-start the same vicious cycle. For example, one of the reasons mercury can be so problematic is that it blocks the very enzymes needed to eliminate it and other heavy metals from the body. Aluminum is particularly damaging to mitochondria, leading to a cascade of inflammatory signals, which then lead to compromised function. There are also a number of combinatory effects that result in exponentially worse outcomes. Glyphosate, for example, not only damages microbiota, mitochondria, and human DNA by itself, but it can also work as a transport agent for aluminum, escorting it through the blood brain barrier to be stored in the brain. Research indicates that elevated levels of aluminum in the brain, among other issues, can contribute to a variety of neurological diseases and neurodegenerative conditions such as Alzheimer's and dementia.

The primary reason binding agents can be such an effective tool is that many of these chemicals, metals, and biotoxin molecules require something to bind to them to neutralize them and escort them out of the body. Without something to bind to, they can get caught in a loop of enterohepatic recirculation, whereby they continue in a cycle of being processed by the liver, carried into the intestines by the bile from the gall bladder, then reabsorbed in the intestines to get processed by the liver again. Binding agents can also act as a major protector for the kidneys by evacuating toxins through the stool instead of being excreted through the urinary tract. By way of their unique chemical structures and electrostatic charges, natural binders can electrically attract, entrap, and escort a wide variety of toxic substances out of the body.

One of the most effective ways to consistently consume binding agents is through your diet. Some plant fibers work as a direct binding agent for toxins, while others work by binding to bile, which helps to escort toxins out of the body that are already bound to bile. Consuming plenty of food-based soluble and insoluble fibers on a regular basis has been found to markedly reduce levels of chemicals, metals, and biotoxins in the body. This is just another reason to include plenty of fruits (particularly the skins) and vegetables in your diet. Pectin, which is found abundantly in apples, cabbage, beets, plums, and the white pith of citrus fruits, is one such fiber that has been shown to be particularly effective at binding to heavy metals and a variety of biotoxins.

The following list contains some of my favorite binders and their particular affinity for various toxic substances. It should be noted that not all products and brands are created equal, and it is worth your due diligence to determine the highest quality brand or product you can find. Because binders have a natural affinity for toxins, purchasing cheap or poorly sourced products may incidentally be contaminated with the very substances you are intending to remove.

— *Chlorella, Spirulina, and Ecklonia Cava:* These three types of algae in particular have been shown to be extremely effective at binding to heavy metals, pesticides, mold toxins, and volatile organic compounds. Beyond their binding capacity, they can also serve as immune modulators and act as a bioavailable source of omega fatty acids and amino acids, which help to transport toxins from deeper tissues into the blood stream. And because these living organisms don't have much of an affinity for essential nutrients and minerals, they can be taken with food and used long-term without risk of nutritional deficiency.

— *Zeolite Clinoptilolite:* Zeolite is a natural clay with an affinity for a broad-spectrum of mold toxins, parasites, endotoxins, pesticides, fluoride, ammonia, mercury, and lead. Research has also demonstrated zeolites' ability to decrease zonulin, the primary molecule that increases gut permeability (leaky gut). Zeolite is a fairly selective binder and has a greater affinity for toxins, but it may bind to some nutrients. It is best to take zeolite on an empty stomach, away from food and other supplements. It is best taken a few weeks at a time before taking a break for a few weeks.

— *Humic and Fulvic Acids:* Humic and fulvic acids are made from decomposed plant material and have been used for thousands of years in Ayurvedic medicine, particularly in the form of shilajit. They have a particular affinity for binding to glyphosate and pesticides, but they also work to improve gut microbial balance and help to increase absorption and transportation of nutrients into cells. Increasing mineral absorption alone can often help in the removal of toxic substances from the body.

— *Activated Charcoal:* Charcoal is probably the most widely known toxin binder on the market. Usually made by exposing plant material like coconut shells or bamboo to an activating agent and high heat, activated charcoal binds to a few mold toxins, pesticides, and biotoxins. Charcoal also has a tendency to bind to nutrients and pharmaceutical drugs as well, so it is best taken on an empty stomach. Charcoal is best not taken for long periods of time. Instead it's best used when an acute toxic exposure or symptom flare occurs.

— *Bentonite Clay:* This clay originates from volcanic ash and has been used for hundreds, if not thousands, of years. While not particularly effective at binding to metals, they can help in neutralizing biotoxins from some molds and other microbes. Clays are best taken a few weeks at a time before taking a break for a few weeks.

— *Silica:* Silica is probably the most effective binder at removing aluminum and thallium from the body. It can be consumed by drinking horsetail tea or by taking any number of silica-based products specifically formulated for binding and detoxification. Silica gels are also commonly used in the case of food poisoning and to bind to endotoxins in the gut, as they have been shown to help restore gastrointestinal balance. Most silica products can be taken for a few weeks before taking a break.

— *Modified Citrus Pectin:* Silica is This slightly modified version of the natural fiber found in citrus fruits is a potent immune modulator and inflammatory reduction agent. It effectively breaks down biofilms and binds mycotoxins and toxic metals, without reducing important minerals like calcium, zinc, selenium, and magnesium. It has also been shown to slow and prevent cancer growth and is safe to take long-term.

Depending on your toxic load, it can be worthwhile to introduce a variety of binders on a regular basis. The most effective method is to focus on sufficient food-based binders found in fruits and vegetable fibers. Adding modified citrus pectin along with specialized algae such as chlorella, spirulina, and Ecklonia cava can make a world of difference over the long-term and carries very little risk. Other natural binders should be taken strategically and always with adequate hydration, as binders tend to act as a bulking agent and slow down bowel transit.

Chapter 7

EXERCISE FOR LONGEVITY

---

*When it comes to health and well-being, regular exercise
is about as close to a magic potion as you can get.*

— THICH NHAT HANH

One of the most memorable moments I have in our travels around the world was a conversation I had with our 35-year-old Airbnb host in Costa Rica. As a tour guide, Javier Armijo has interacted with numerous travelers from Europe and the United States. While discussing the tourists he works with, he said, "The first thing I noticed, for kids especially, is that they are not as active. They don't know how to even move. Something very simple like getting into the kayak becomes a 30-second task, while kids here at the age of five or six are already climbing trees and getting their fruit. When it comes to something more complicated, like coming out of the truck even, they just have odd motion. I don't know how to say it . . . With the simple tasks, they are not acting like kids." On one hand, this didn't surprise me a great deal. In the age of video games, the Internet, and digital technology, his observations are somewhat expected. But as someone from a culture with an abundance of these modern technologies, I guess I just hadn't noticed how bad it has become. He was able to see the sharp contrast between local kids and foreigners in such a profound way, and it is very telling of the state of exercise and movement in many industrialized cultures.

Over the last 60 years in the U.S., and especially in the last 20, we've become more accustomed to the indoor environment. More of our work is done inside, sitting on the computer. And fewer people have jobs that involve any semblance of physical activity. The manual labor of a century ago has now been outsourced to automated machines. For the first time in history, because of the increase in sedentary work, time for exercise must be set aside and placed on the schedule.

This certainly wasn't the case for the elders throughout their life. When I asked them about exercise, I honestly felt a bit silly. Just observing the way their society currently operates was enough for me to know the answer before I even asked the question. Sixty years ago in many of the villages, there were few roads and no cars. In Costa Rica, horseback and horse-drawn carts were used for extremely long treks, but for the most part, they walked everywhere. It wasn't uncommon to walk 25 miles a day or more.

Michelino Scudu of Sardinia spoke about his 55-mile treks as a shepherd. "I worked a lot and walked a lot too. Along with my flock, I did the seasonal herding from the Gennargentu to the coast on foot! Like animals! Loaded with bags," he said as he laughed. "Being a shepherd is a very hard job." Walking was far and away the most common form of exercise over the course of the elders' lives.

As children, they kept busy with sports and play. But as they grew into their teen years and adulthood, they had little concept of leisure and there was no exercising for fun. As adults, the elders' life was consumed by movement and exercise, as it served a productive purpose. At age 91, Jose Santos of Guanacaste said, "No, we didn't have exercise. Exercise was work. I know of it, but I never liked it. My work was in the fields with the machete and planting crops like Roma beans." I couldn't help but laugh when he said, "I know of it," when asked about exercise. They didn't think about movement in terms of staying fit. Physical activity was required to get things done. Orestis Portelos of Ikaria said the same thing:

"When you are doing these kinds of jobs, you have no free time to do anything else. One needs to take care of the oxen, the mules, the gardens, the vineyards."

Whether it was walking to work, tending the garden, building a fence, herding sheep or cattle from one place to the next, or walking two kilometers to the river to wash clothes, exercise was coupled with survival and daily necessities. Everybody contributed based on their capacity to do so. Men did more of the heavy lifting and physically demanding work. Women tended to work longer hours around the house, in the garden, raising kids, preparing food, and holding everything together. If children weren't at school or playing, you'd often find them helping the family in the gardens and orchards. Their whole life was movement. At 104 years old, Giulio Podda of Sardinia recalled a time that he and a team of three others used to load 50,000 to 60,000 pounds of salt into wagons every day. "In Macchiareddu, I was a wagon worker. I loaded twenty-cubic-meter wagons. It was no fun, eh," he said as he laughed.

Almost every aspect of their life included movement, and most of it was done outside during daylight hours. Without electricity, they did very little work indoors after the sun went down. I also got the distinct sense that they did not rush to get things done, as there were few deadlines. Yet they seem to have a very good work ethic, making sure to continue to progress with their work. I think 94-year-old Salvatore Scanu of Sardinia said it best: "When I was younger, the body was busy and the mind was still. Now what I see is that the mind is busy and the body is still. I think that's a real problem."

THE BENEFITS OF EXERCISE

The longevity benefits of exercise and movement have long been touted by researchers and media outlets alike. In fact, you'd probably have a hard time finding anybody who disagrees with the idea that exercise is beneficial for health. I suspect the profound benefits of exercise are likely still underappreciated. Sure, we'd all like to be able to jog into old age without aches and pains. While the right type of movement serves an important role in maintaining mobility into old age, it serves many other important roles in maintaining health. Far from just improving cardiovascular health, metabolic health, and body composition, there is no organ or system that doesn't benefit either directly or indirectly from adequate and appropriate exercise.

Improved Immune Function

One major benefit of exercise that flies under the radar is the impact it has on overall immune function. Immune system dysfunctions have increased markedly in the United States over the past 30 years for a variety of reasons. Common infections prove to be a greater threat to the elderly. Exercise is one of the methods we have at our disposal to protect against this. Many warn of overexercising when you're ill or battling severe chronic dysfunction, and this is valid. If the nervous system is overburdened and lacks resources to respond to exercise, then inflammation may increase. But consistent exercise is also very beneficial for balancing and improving immune tolerance. Exercise improves regulatory T-cell activity, improves vagal tone, increases gut microbiota diversity, and improves the gut and brain barriers.

Improved Brain Function

Another long-term benefit of exercise is at the level of the brain. Because of increasing rates of Alzheimer's and dementia, it's become common to accept that brain function will quickly deteriorate as you age beyond your 70s. In fact, this is the one of the biggest fears about reaching old age. But what if you don't have to lose your memory? What if exercise could help you remain sharp as a tack beyond 100?

With exercise comes an increased production of nitric oxide synthase, growth hormone, serotonin, dopamine, and a tiny protein called brain-derived neurotrophic factor (BDNF), which all play major roles in keeping you mentally sharp. Research has shown that exercise increases neuroplasticity, increases neuronal synapse efficiency, fortifies existing neuronal networks, increases focus, improves mood, improves sleep, and reduces your risk of neurodegeneration. Other than sleep and perhaps meditation, exercise might be the most brain-protective health habit in which you can engage. And according to research, the greater the exercise intensity, the greater the neuroprotective effects—so long as you don't overtrain.

Improved Mitochondrial Function

At the cellular level, exercise proves critical for healthy mitochondrial function. And healthy mitochondria are critical for efficient energy production, reduced cellular damage, and harmonious epigenetic expression in all cells. This is the primary reason exercise has such a profound impact on mitochondrion-dense organs such as the brain and heart. When you engage in intense exercise and provide a healthy stress to your mitochondria, they may struggle to make enough energy to meet the demand. In response, they will activate a process known as mitochondrial biogenesis. This process is a form of self-replication and works to increase mitochondrial mass in order to boost cellular energy and efficiency. As you adapt to make new, healthy mitochondria, your cells have an increased capacity to handle stress and carry out essential functions throughout the body. Charalampos Kratzas of Ikaria encapsulated this idea well when he said, "The work I was doing contributed most to my health. The more you sit, the easier the job you are doing, the less you live. The harder you work, the tougher you are."

HOW WE THINK ABOUT FITNESS

When we look at a fitness model or another person perceived to be in great shape, they tend to have a certain amount of muscle mass or definition. In the West, this has become the ideal look for health and wellness. For as much exercise as the elders did throughout their life, they indicated they were never particularly muscular or looked "fit" in the terms we might think of, nor were the current 30- to 60-year-old locals that I saw. This modern, Western concept of what it means to be fit or in shape generally emphasizes aesthetics over function. It really says nothing about the health of a person on the inside.

To contradict myself a bit, however, I did notice an obvious trend over the years as a practitioner running blood, hormone, and metabolic tests for my clients. Clients who exercised regularly and ate a fairly poor diet usually had better markers on lab tests than clients who ate more consciously and did not exercise. To be clear, however, an outside appearance of "health"—having 6 percent body fat and six-pack abs—absolutely does not confer true inner health. There are too many other lifestyle factors that determine health and longevity beyond low body-fat percentage.

Hormetic Stress

It is important to keep in mind that most exercise results in added stress to the body. So when it comes to optimal health and longevity, the way to think about most forms of exercise is as a hormetic stress. Hormetic stress is sort of like saying a little poison is healthy but a lot is dangerous. It is a biological characteristic whereby a low-level stress or damage can invoke a favorable adaptive response that results in a more resilient or adaptable trait. If, however, you consistently exercise beyond your ability to recover, you will do more harm than good. There is a sweet spot when it comes to intense exercise and movement. And this sweet spot has everything to do with your sleep, health state, lifestyle practices, diet, and exercise frequency.

Hormetic stress, or hormesis, is an important concept that probably doesn't get the attention it deserves. The profound benefit of hormetic stress is that it helps make you more antifragile. It improves long-term resiliency in the face of adversity. With the right amount of perceived environmental stress, coupled with a subsequent phase of necessary repair, you are able to fully recover from the stress signal. This will result in greater resiliency, allowing for greater adaptation and coherent response to future perceived environmental pressures.

The most obvious example is strength training. By placing your musculoskeletal system under intense and repeated stress with weights, a little tissue damage occurs. With enough damage, exhaustion and soreness is a notable symptom in the following days. But as the musculoskeletal system repairs and recovers, it adapts by building more strength and/or endurance to deal with the environmental conditions. Continue this incremental process of increased stress, damage, and recovery, and you'll continue to grow more muscle and improve resiliency. However, with too much stress or too little recovery, the result is no growth and no added resiliency. Push too hard and you can even decrease resiliency.

This concept is not relegated to only muscle growth. It applies to many cellular processes and systems in the body as well, including the mind. Navy SEALs are extremely antifragile in both body and mind because they have progressively adapted to greater and greater levels of perceived stress. A few other examples of hormetic stressors include ultraviolet radiation from the sun, environmental microbes, extreme temperatures, atmospheric pressure, low oxygen levels, and phytochemicals from plant foods.

Exercise creates a stimulus, and the body produces an adaptive response. Without adequate recovery, you're likely adding stress to the body. And unfortunately, all stresses are cumulative. Whether it's mental, emotional, chemical, physical, or electromagnetic stress, it all enters the same pot. We can't isolate the stresses in the body. And because of the many forms of stress in today's modern world, particularly mental and emotional stress, many people exercise as a way to cope with these stressors. And this may be problematic. The art is figuring out how much total stress you can put on your system so that you're creating a healthy response and not breaking down the body further.

Heart Rate Variability

There is a certain level of mindfulness when it comes to exercise and its relation to overall health and longevity. One of the better ways you can determine your body's real-time capacity for exercise stress is by tracking your heart rate variability (HRV). There are many devices that you can use to easily track HRV on a daily basis. Heart rate variability measures the frequency variation of your heart beats. Generally speaking, the higher the variation, the greater the balance of your autonomic nervous system, and the more your body is ready for exercise.

Using HRV measurements can also be a great way to get to know your body as you feel the subtle differences associated with high and low HRV. This can be done without the use of technology as well, as you feel into and get to know your system—gauging when your body and mind don't have much capacity, when you truly feel rested, and how much exertion you can handle without tipping the scales. Where most people fail in this equation is not getting enough restorative sleep and rest.

Of course the elders had no way of tracking HRV in their life. And they didn't really have the luxury of adjusting their workload based on how they felt. Work had to get done no matter what. While many of them worked quite hard, their other lifestyle stressors were quite low, and they got the sleep equation correct.

CHOOSING THE RIGHT EXERCISE FOR YOU

People in the modern world now have an abundance of choices about how to move and which activities to engage in. This has resulted in a variety of exercise trends that have come and gone throughout the years, creating confusion about which form of exercise is best. Many people have an idea of fitness in their mind. But the question you should be asking yourself is, "Fit for what?" The definition of optimal fitness may differ if you are a collegiate athlete, competitive marathon runner, CrossFit games competitor, firefighter, farmer, accountant, or stay-at-home parent to three little ones. If your objective is to add muscle mass, the strategies you employ to accomplish this will be drastically different than if your objective is to qualify for the Boston Marathon. Neither may be effective if your ultimate objective is optimal health and longevity.

There are many researchers trying to get a handle on how much and what type of exercises are best for longevity. It shouldn't surprise you that there is no meaningful consensus. I suspect there never will be. The lifetime of a human incorporates far too much movement to study. Of course, we're all unique. Research continues to show that there are tremendous benefits to all forms and intensities of exercise and movement. The key is figuring out which form will benefit you most at this point in your life and how much to do.

There are some who suggest that the best form of exercise is the one you will do consistently long-term. There is a lot to be said for the sentiment in this recommendation. Doing exercise you enjoy is certainly better than exercise you hate. I also want to offer that if you continue to engage in an exercise that is throwing your system out of balance, causing you physical pain, complication, or suffering in any way, the better solution is to stop and find something that will help bring more balance. I've seen this situation arise with long-distance runners, weight lifters, boxers, and cyclists to name a few. Sometimes there are ways to make the activity more harmonious so that one can continue to enjoy it. Sometimes you just have to know when to call it quits.

There is a word of caution that comes with modern approaches to exercise. Many strategies tend to restrict or isolate movement patterns. If you get locked into one style of exercise or movement pattern over long periods, you run the risk of increasing your chance of injury or creating imbalance. Depending on your current context and objectives, you can determine which activities are best. Over the years, your goals will likely shift. The key is to use a wide variety of movement and exercise strategies throughout your life as appropriate, just like the elders did naturally. If the goal is healthy aging, we need to reframe our perspective on exercise and accept that there's not one single most effective strategy for everyone at every point in their life.

There is also the mental/emotional aspect to exercise. Humans aren't robots. There is tremendous value in finding activities that are either productive or fun. You can mow your lawn with a reel mower instead of hiring somebody to cut your grass with a gas-powered mower that creates excess noise and air pollution. You can paint your house or landscape your yard. Actively playing with your dog or your children is another great way to move. Playing basketball, tennis, or golf or swimming are fantastic ways to get exercise. The ultimate goal should be to find sources of movement and activity that give you joy and keep you coming back for more, without causing imbalance.

One thing is certain, 30 minutes of exercise each day isn't enough to compensate for 23.5 sedentary hours. The key to long-term health and longevity is consistent movement each day, in a variety of ways throughout life.

Functional Mobility and Corrective Exercise

In the past decade, there has been an explosion in functional mobility training in Western societies. Generally, functional exercises focus on training your musculoskeletal system and nervous system through various movement patterns that improve balance, mobility, strength, and core stability. The lack of daily functional movement created by sedentary lifestyles has undoubtedly created a greater need to incorporate more functional mobility training.

Within this category, you'll find many popular practices such as CrossFit, yoga, Pilates, and others that also cross into high-intensity interval training (HIIT), strength training, and steady-state cardio. Beyond these popular methods, there are numerous independent outlets that provide specific mobility work designed to improve your muscular and structural balance, joint and soft tissue integrity, and range of motion.

Because of the imbalances created by modern lifestyles, functional mobility training and corrective exercise are some of the greatest tools at your disposal for creating a more aligned, balanced, and coherent musculoskeletal system at any age. This process should ideally be assisted by a professional who can assess your imbalances and guide you into proper training methods to improve function, reassert balance, and reduce the total-body stress burden.

High-Intensity Interval Training

High-intensity interval training (HIIT) has become quite popular in the United States, particularly for those looking to lose body fat and maintain muscle mass. These are cardiovascular workouts that combine short bursts of all-out, intense exercise with subsequent periods of rest or very low-intensity movement. Research shows HIIT is one of the most time-efficient ways to lose excess fat, increase muscle, increase maximal aerobic capacity, increase testosterone, boost brain derived-neurotrophic factor (BDNF), improve mitochondrial function, and lower your resting heart rate. However, most people should limit this type of training to two to three times a week in order to provide adequate rest and recovery. If you have significant health issues or challenges with mobility, HIIT might be reduced further or avoided completely.

Resistance Training

Resistance or strength exercises are a great way to build muscle mass and increase strength. There are significant benefits for all genders and ages who engage in at least some resistance training. Whether you use weights, bands, your own body weight, or another form of resistance, regularly incorporating strength training will help maintain muscle mass, improve bone health, reduce excess fat, boost growth hormone, improve balance, improve cardiovascular health, and improve hormonal balance. The more resistance training you do in a day, the more recovery you'll need before your next bout. In general, for adults, two to three days per week of moderate strength training for 30 to 45 minutes is sufficient for long-term health and well-being.

Steady-State Cardio

This form of exercise can be accomplished by doing yard work, manual labor, sporting activities, or going for a jog. Anything that consistently elevates your heart rate in a low to moderate way for 20 to 60 minutes or more should be considered. This is a great way to improve cardiovascular health and metabolic function without worrying about muscle mass or significant fatigue.

For most people, steady-state cardio can be done regularly without the need for much rest and recovery. The caution here is in doing any particular movement repetitively and for long periods of time. This may eventually introduce musculoskeletal imbalances and increase sympathetic (stress) activation in the body if countervailing movements aren't also incorporated to establish structural and soft tissue balance.

Yin Movement

This is a bit of a foreign concept to many people in Western cultures because we tend to be dominated by yang energy. Among the many attributes of yang energy is the idea of a forceful, active, fast, loud, and outward expression. The U.S. culture is highly dominated by yang energy, and the way we typically exercise mirrors this cultural expression.

Yin energy, on the other hand, is the opposite, expressing a soft, still, slow, quiet, and inward expression. By incorporating yin movements into your routine, you're able to gain a great deal of benefit from moving without adding additional stress to the body. The subtle movement and energy flow throughout the body increases your overall energy and improves your ability to repair.

My friend Paul Chek, a corrective and high-performance exercise kinesiologist, calls this type of movement *working in*, drawing a distinction from working out. Some of the oldest known practices, such as yin yoga, tai chi, tao yin, and qigong, incorporate various yin movements. In contrast with most other forms of yoga, yin yoga is a more passive and slow practice where some poses are held for five minutes or more, offering deeper access to the fascia, connective tissue, and joints.

You can also apply your own yin movements in your daily life. For example, you can do body squats, joint mobility drills, walk, or anything else you can think of to move your body. The general rule of thumb is to focus your awareness on your breath and move slowly and softly enough so as not to increase your rate of breathing. You should be able to maintain a soft breath through the nose as you go. If you feel the need to breathe through your mouth, you're working too hard.

Cultivating a practice of yin movement will bring greater balance and harmony to the energy systems of your body. These movements will also help increase awareness to the benefits of slowing down in many areas of your life that rarely get a break. For people dominated by fast-paced yang energy, yin movements will bring nourishing energy into the body, facilitating greater healing capacity, increased subtle awareness, and improved well-being.

Walking

Without a doubt, walking is the most underutilized, universal, and effective form of movement that you can incorporate. There are mounds of research espousing the benefits walking has on overall health. Even a 30-minute walk at a normal walking pace helps improve digestion, improves blood sugar control, and increases lymphatic flow. This simple activity puts very low stress on the body and is the safest mode of exercise for those with health issues, injuries, and musculoskeletal imbalances. If one activity were most associated with longevity, it would be walking.

If your average day includes very little activity, you should aim for five to seven hours of walking per week. If you incorporate other forms of exercise on a regular basis, you may want to set aside just an hour per day for low-intensity walking on your rest days.

KEEP MOVING

One of the most noticeable lifestyle differences I found was between retirement in the United States and retirement in cultures of the elders around the world. Even if the elders formally stopped working for pay, their mindsets around work hardly shifted. They often continued beyond their 80s, working around the house, in the vegetable gardens, taking care of animals, and tending to the land.

At 91 years old, Jose Santos of Guanacaste said he mostly relaxes but continues to have some fun working on his property: "We still have little pieces of land, and I get to clear it out a bit with the machete—planting a little corn for our daily use."

In Okinawa, I met Fuji Sasaki at his office, where he still ran a company that employs upward of 200 people. Fuji was 85 years old and said he has no plans of retiring anytime soon. "I think I am going to continue my businesses maybe until I finish my life," he said as he excitedly laughed. This was similar to the mentality expressed by Hideko Kamida as well. Hideko was one of the most remarkable people we met in Okinawa. At 97, she managed her house and large garden on her own and had no intention of slowing down. She planned on working until the end. Hideko had absolutely no trouble tilling her soil by hand, using her *kama* (sickle) to cut the sugarcane, harvesting her vegetables each season, and picking fruits from her trees. Hideko's daughter told me she caught her mom climbing one of her orange trees to pick fruit two years prior, when Hideko was 95. Every so often she would walk to her friend's house, a mile and a half down the road. In Okinawa, she was the epitome of what they call *genki*—very lively and energetic. I couldn't get enough time with Hideko. She just blew us all away.

One of the more fascinating gentlemen I got to know in Ikaria was Georgios Stenos. Georgios began keeping bees at the age of 18 because he read how useful bees are for the planet. He continued to the day I met him at the age of 85, with no plans to stop. He estimated that he's been stung thousands of times over the years and doesn't even feel the stings anymore. According to him, you'll never find a beekeeper who has arthritis or rheumatism of any kind because the bee venom stimulates a strong immune system. I told him that scientific research agrees with his assertion, as bee venom therapy has been used for thousands of years and continues to demonstrate amazing healing effects today in a number of conditions. His beekeeping is a perfect example of hormetic stress. Along with his bees, Georgios took care of his extensive vegetable garden, where he grew most of the food he eats.

Then there is Okinawan resident Tatsuo Kakinohana, who officially retired from his government job at 64 years old. At 82, he had taken up several hobbies that occupied his time and kept him moving. Not only did he restore classic cars as his primary hobby, he wrote calligraphy and had been learning to play the ukulele as part of a band with his friends.

Despite their age, the elders understood that moving and engaging with life is an important part of their senior years. They very much felt like they had something to offer and had a passion to live the remainder of their life with zest. Without TVs, computers, casinos, and many of the fruitless, inactive trappings of the modern world, they didn't get sucked into a passive existence. Even at the senior care center in Okinawa, there was a firm intent to incorporate movement, dance, and karaoke into their days. The residents watched and participated in entertaining skits and dances on stage that had the whole room bursting with laughter.

For each of the elders, with old age came physical deterioration and a slowing down. But despite their pace, they kept moving, determined not to let their hindered pace get in the way of continuing to live. Watching 99-year-old Michelino Scudu slowly pedal his stationary bike—and 91-year-old Vitalio Melis's hampered jog as he left our interview—demonstrated that with old age comes a restriction of movement and a modified perspective. Despite any physical limitations, most of the elders moved without a great deal of pain. They adjusted with grace to a new way of being that still allowed them to enjoy the most important aspects of life. For Giulio Podda, it was riding his bike and whittling wood. After I was done visiting with him, he gifted me a wooden mallet he had carved, then demonstrated his bike-riding skills as he did a slow and wobbly lap down the street and back. I was stunned. Not bad for 104 years old.

MOVE TO THRIVE

There are so many forms of exercise and movement that *can* be beneficial to your overall health. I invite you to let your unique circumstances and condition guide the best path forward for you. That said, there are a handful of opportunities that are available to just about everyone, no matter their age, when it comes to using movement to improve health and well-being.

Correct the Imbalance

If you're looking to engage with the most optimal form of movement and exercise for you, the first place to begin is to bring awareness to the current condition of your body. Where are your structural imbalances and misalignments? Which muscles are tight or loose? Where do you lack mobility or stability? How much capacity does your nervous system have to deal with exercise stress?

In order to maximize coherence in the body, you need to get a sense for what needs correction. Finding a skilled coach or practitioner may prove extremely valuable if you have the means. I've been impressed by the ability of many certified Chek practitioners (www.chekinstitute.com), who are specialists in corrective exercise and high-performance kinesiology. There are many others who can properly assess the state of your body and guide you into balance.

Ditch the Shoes

There are tremendous benefits that come from stepping back into your feet. Going barefoot has shown to reduce anxiety and stress, alter brainwave patterns, and balance neurotransmitter levels. The structural integrity of your feet also play an incredibly important role in how the rest of your musculoskeletal structure is aligned. Not only will you benefit from improved strength and integrity of your feet and ankles, barefoot movement also facilitates greater dexterity, balance, posture, proprioception, and mechanics.

In addition, there are a number of reflex points on the bottom of the feet that get stimulated naturally and increase harmony and the natural healing processes of many organs and systems. Interacting directly with the earth allows for an exchange of electric charge, reducing excess inflammation and creating greater coherence in your entire system.

Take a Walk

There is little downside to walking. Whatever you can do to increase the number of steps you take in a day will subtly and profoundly work in your favor over the course of your life.

Diversity of Movement

Combining a wide range of intensity, duration, and styles of movement throughout your life will help protect against physical imbalance and repetitive injury. By taking advantage of the benefits of many forms of movement, you improve the health of your nervous system, cardiovascular system, and musculoskeletal system with good mobility into your later years.

Dance and Play

If elective activity is all work and no play, you're missing some of the most profound benefits available to you. Dance and play have been shown to dramatically improve mental/emotional well-being, as they allow you to express creativity and emotion through embodied, somatic movements and social engagement.

Resistance for Youth

As we get older, sarcopenia, or the gradual loss of muscle mass, inevitably occurs due to natural hormonal decline and loss of function in the body. Even mild but consistent application of resistance training can work to slow down the process of muscle loss. Resistance training and high-intensity training are also the greatest ways to stimulate the production of hormones such as testosterone and growth hormone that keep you young. High-intensity training also has a wonderful ability to stimulate the growth of new mitochondria, which is one of the most important things that you can do to maintain youthful function at the cellular level.

Movement Snacks

As we continue to see the reduction in the need for manual labor in the workplace, we have an opportunity to reframe our ideas about movement. Instead of dedicating one block of time each day to movement, you can find ways to incorporate movement and activity throughout your day. As my friend and founder of Primal Play, Darryl Edwards, says, "It's more beneficial to incorporate movement snacks throughout the day instead of eating one big meal." Whether it's 30 seconds, two minutes, or a half hour, look for ways to consciously engage in more movement. If you just take notice, you'll find so many opportunities throughout your day to take the stairs, park farther away, walk and balance on a curb, do a few push-ups, stretch, move heavy objects, play with the dog, and the like.

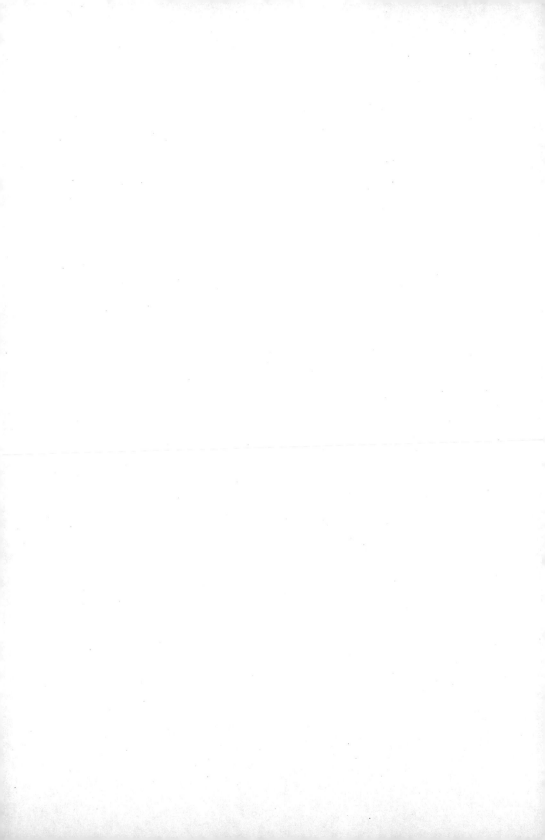

Chapter 8

PROCESSING STUCK EMOTION

Adverse childhood experiences are the single greatest
unaddressed public health threat facing our nation today.

— DR. ROBERT BLOCK, FORMER PRESIDENT OF
THE AMERICAN ACADEMY OF PEDIATRICS

Whenever I'm asked about the longevity cultures and their ways of life, there are two main questions that always seem to surface. Most people want to know about their diets, perhaps not surprisingly. The other question often relates to what about their way of life surprised me most. And what surprised me most was how much impact the village pace of life had on my sense of well-being. The relaxed and easeful energy was quite profound.

Furthermore, in listening to the elders speak about childhood, their family life, and how they were raised, it was abundantly clear that, as kids, they perceived more safety, security, connection, and acceptance, and dealt with far less trauma than what is experienced in most modern industrial societies. They undoubtedly dealt with hardship, overwhelming experiences, and trauma just as all other children around the world might. It is an inevitable part of the human experience. While I have no real way of quantifying or qualifying the elders' childhood experiences with any real certainty, I suspect that they had little to none of the types of early childhood trauma and attachment disorders that are so rampant in modern society.

The greatest health education I ever received were the years I focused solely on my health practice and was regularly working one-on-one with clients. The uniqueness in each person was unbelievably apparent and each personal story taught me something new. As I became more educated and skilled at guiding my clients to better health, I also became more skilled at recognizing the missing pieces. There came a point where I was quite confident in my ability to give my clients the information, strategies, and plan to help them feel great. Yet there were always a handful of clients that wouldn't implement the plan I laid out.

At first, it frustrated me to no end. Every client was referred by word-of-mouth, as I didn't advertise my services. I couldn't understand why somebody would seek me out, pay a bunch of money, and not follow through with what I gave them. Because I truly cared about them, I devoted more of my time and energy, trying to motivate and inspire them. But it didn't make much difference.

Then one day it all just clicked. These clients that I cared about and was dedicated to helping were quite literally incapable of following through, no matter what I did, because I was incapable of guiding them to what they really needed. We were working on improving balance and coherence in the realm of everything conscious. What they really needed was improving alignment and coherence in the realm of the subconscious. My clients were unable to see the real aspects that were blocking them from healing, and I was blind to them as well. When I started to learn how to see, an entire new world opened up—one I had little clue as to how to navigate.

ADVERSE CHILDHOOD EXPERIENCES

In 1998, the Centers for Disease Control and Prevention (CDC) and Kaiser Permanente conducted the Adverse Childhood Experience (ACE) study. They surveyed more than 17,000 adults, asking if they recall facing any of 10 challenging experiences in childhood. They labeled these *adverse childhood experiences* (ACEs) and included such notable instances as parental divorce, physical/sexual/emotional abuse, neglect, substance abuse by parents, domestic violence in the family, or parents getting incarcerated.

The researchers found some shocking correlations that forced them to rethink behavioral psychology. On average, the adults that reported a large number of ACEs demonstrated a major increased risk of at least 7 of the top 10 causes of death. For those who reported six ACEs, the data indicated a 20-year reduction in lifespan, on average, compared to those who reported zero ACEs. There were increases in depression, autoimmune disorders, cancer, and even risk of suicide associated with increased ACEs. Now, correlation doesn't necessarily indicate causation. But the statistical data was overwhelming, revealing the notion that something deeper was going on and it needed to be investigated further.

There have been numerous other investigative studies that have corroborated these findings and explored them further. They all demonstrate the same thing—there are overwhelming experiences that we all face in childhood that have the ability to negatively influence our physical and mental health in profound ways.

One of the obvious explanations that researchers were quick to investigate was the strong possibility that these adverse childhood events could simply cause severe patterns of unhealthy behavior—things such as smoking, alcoholism, or drug use. And perhaps it was merely the chronic, unhealthy behavior that caused the statistical increase of ill-effects and shorter lives. But when they adjusted for the behavioral component, the data remained consistent. Even those who weren't smokers, drinkers, or drug users still showed a similar increased risk for chronic disease.

The researchers of the ACE study estimate that roughly two-thirds of the United States population has at least one ACE, and one out of every eight has at least four ACEs. From a purely correlative perspective, these numbers seem to paint a fairly accurate picture of the nation's illness crisis. And what is even more revelatory is the recognition that the ACE study is only able to capture an incomplete snapshot of an individual's traumatic life experiences. It is no fault of the study design, of course. Most of us simply can't recall any experiences before we are two or three years old or even older.

There is another challenge with any attempt to accurately record ACEs through conscious memory. More often than you might expect, an individual who experiences a very significant trauma will completely forget about it. It is almost as if it didn't exist. The pain of an experience can be so severe that the mind buries it to avoid any conscious recall. And the final notable challenge with accurately recording ACEs is the near impossibility of assessing what should be classified as an adverse event and qualitatively determining the effects. For example, if my third-grade teacher mocked me in front of the entire class because I was a poor reader, can we classify this as a traumatic event? What if it happened weekly? Or perhaps I was bullied and picked on all year in fourth grade—does this count? Things get very fuzzy, and it becomes difficult to accurately represent an individual's overwhelming life experiences.

Despite the challenges of documenting adverse childhood events, the ACE study has shed enormous light on the relationship between early childhood trauma and adult illness. There is only one way to document and record all the painful and traumatic experiences you have faced in life. They have all been etched in your subconscious mind and sometimes crystallized in your body systems—that is, until they get transformed or processed and integrated.

BIOLOGY OF THE SUBCONSCIOUS

From the perspective of mainstream Western medicine in the United States, the manifestation of chronic disease in the physical body can really only be caused by something in the physical world. The doctor may suspect the cause is poor diet or lack of exercise or unlucky genetics or even job stress. It is commonly taught that the physical world is the only acceptable reason for the manifestation of chronic health issues. There is a big elephant in the room, though, in the unacknowledged power of the subconscious.

When medical research is performed on humans, the researchers openly acknowledge that a double-blind, placebo-controlled study design is the gold standard. Why? Because the placebo effect can skew the data if sufficient measures aren't taken to prevent it. Basically, people's subconscious expectations can cause them to show an improvement, even when they're not receiving a "real" treatment. What's even more ironic, some of the researchers who use this study design continue to deny that the placebo effect can play a role in healing. But at this point it is clear. Research on the placebo effect has demonstrated that an individual's intention, expectation, or belief can absolutely result in physical healing, even if the substance or procedure is inert.

On the flip side is the nocebo effect. Your expectation or belief that a substance will cause an undesired or negative effect can absolutely generate such an effect, despite the inert nature of the substance. This means that with your awareness, you have the ability to create change and healing in the body, as well as the ability to generate physical symptoms and remain stuck in disharmony. Educators and authors such as Lynne McTaggart, Joe Dispenza, Bruce Lipton, and John Sarno have even centered much of their work around mind/body illnesses and the profound healing potential that exists through intention and awareness.

A large majority of your past experiences are recorded as subconscious information, emotional charge, and energetic distortion that may get crystalized in the body's neurobiology and epigenetic expression. The stored information, emotions, and energies are subjective interpretations of past experiences. In this way, the body acts as a reflected, life-long, archival record of perceived experiences.

Your mind, then, tends to filter current experiences through the colored lens of past perceptions that have been stored in the subconscious (a.k.a. your body). This means your subconscious mind is running programmed neurobiological patterns and expressing genes based on the past. It's why two people could have essentially the same experience but their body systems respond in completely different fashions. Perceptions and beliefs from the past tend to create your existing reality today. These perceptions and beliefs will also predict your future reality—unless you transform or process what's stuck and change the subconscious programs that guide epigenetic expression.

Current experience —> subconscious mind / past perceptions —> epigenetic expression —> conscious interpretation of current experience

According to Bruce Lipton, the subconscious mind may be processing 1 million times more information than the conscious mind. And unlike your conscious mind, the subconscious doesn't make mistakes. It keeps a perfect record and reflects it in the body systems. It is up to us to learn how to interpret the divine communication of our own body.

When I opened up to the idea that the calcified nodules and knee pain I experienced from 13 years old until 35 years old had a subconscious component, I was finally able to resolve the issue. It was Carl Jung who wisely stated, "Until you make the unconscious conscious, it will direct your life and you will call it fate." I wish I had been able to recognize this truth earlier in life. The repeated messages of pain and physical deformity were there all along. I just wasn't able to consciously understand what my body was really saying.

The body is always communicating through biological patterns of information—sometimes subtle, other times not so subtle. It could show up as chronic knee pain or it could show up as chronically elevated blood pressure, anxiety, or cancer. It is only through the filter of the conscious mind that you may misinterpret these patterned messages.

I was working with a client who was convinced his skin inflammation was fundamentally caused by imbalances in his gut microbiota. A previous practitioner had run tests that absolutely showed imbalances and what appeared to be yeast overgrowth. I asked him why he thought his gut ecosystem was out of balance. He admitted that he didn't always eat the best foods and implement healthy habits. He knew what he *should* be eating, and he did want to feel better. So why wasn't he following through with his healthy lifestyle? We figured out it was primarily because he didn't feel worthy and accepted. He didn't feel like he was enough. This subconscious pattern of beliefs influenced his behavior and his biology. His mind was conditioned despite the fact that he had an extremely "normal" childhood that didn't include any glaring traumatic events.

SUBCONSCIOUS PROGRAMS

The various processes and distinct stages of childhood development are anything but arbitrary. Each stage plays a necessary role in laying down the templates of biological function and behavioral expression that orient and keep the child safe in the world. Whether it is temperature fluctuations, food, sound, light, environmental microbes, or the attentiveness to a child's needs by caretakers, everything the child senses works to influence thoughts, behavior, and epigenetic expression. An infant child is the very definition of an open system, absorbing and adapting to all energetic stimuli.

Until an infant reaches approximately 18 to 24 months old, the child's brain primarily operates in the slowest recorded human brain-wave cycle, ranging from 0.5 to 4 hertz, known as delta waves. This state is associated with rejuvenation and growth in the body. In adulthood, brain activity dominated by delta waves is typically only produced during deep sleep, the moment before death, and in very advanced meditators during meditation. Nearly all the information taken in by the child during this stage bypasses the conscious mind without judgment or bias and is directly downloaded to the unconscious mind. It is also theorized that the delta state allows access to the universal mind and the collective unconscious. This unconscious, "brain-dead" state is part of the reason why it is so difficult to consciously remember anything prior to two years old.

From two to six years of age, the child's brain operates mostly in the theta brain wave state. Creativity and inspiration are often generated from a theta brain wave state, along with insight, imagination, spiritual connection, healing, and growth. This is the realm of the subconscious mind and is associated with deep relaxation, REM sleep, and hypnosis. When the brain is operating in theta, the mind is open to suggestion and capable of immense learning. And it is in this state where most of the mind's deep-seated subconscious programs reside.

So for the first six years of life, a child is primarily in a hypnotic trance. Without much discrimination or discernment, the child absorbs a myriad of subconscious beliefs and programs based on her perceptions of the world or to those given to her. And through this programmed process, the child begins to generate functional awareness that allows for self-consciousness. These subconscious beliefs and programs will form the baseline templates of biological function and behavioral expression into adulthood unless they are reprogrammed.

In these first six years of life it is immensely critical for the child to *feel* unconditionally loved, appreciated, safe, supported, validated, accepted, and worthy on a consistent basis. If, as young children, we constantly perceive and adopt limiting beliefs, disconnection, low self-worth, or lack of safety, these subconscious programs generate patterns of thoughts, emotions, behaviors, and genetic expression to both create a sense of safety and generate a reality that matches the perceptions and beliefs. For example, if an emotionally sensitive child is constantly scolded by her primary caregiver who tells her, "Stop crying! Don't be so sensitive!" her subconscious story will likely be something along the lines of, "I am not loved for who I am. I'm not okay. I must shut down a part of me in order to receive love. I am bad and wrong, and I need to improve." In response, the child learns to stop processing emotion in front of the caregiver—and perhaps stop processing them all together. Her immune regulation may change, and she may develop any number of chronic conditions. Something similar to this hypothetical example is likely the norm in the United States—not the exception.

One of the primary mechanisms that humans use to learn social skills is through mirror neurons. As children and adults, we have sets of neurons that are specifically dedicated to emulating the behavior of others. In this way, we are able to learn the intention and emotion of others, not through thinking and reasoning, but through imitating and feeling. If our parents exhibit a high level of compassion and patience, even at a year old, we can better understand compassion and patience because of mirror neurons. Likewise, if we have anxious or angry parents, the mirror neurons may tend to foster similar behavior. And from my experience, there are also other, more subtle energetic mechanisms through which we learn these behaviors, emotions, and energies. But this is my experience, nothing scientific that I am aware of.

In adulthood, mirror neurons remain active and extremely sensitive, picking up even the slightest facial cues and micro-expressions when we communicate. We then mirror the micro-expression of others so we can better understand the emotions they are communicating. It's as if we can understand and imprint the expression and emotion through our body as it copies theirs. In fact, one of the unintended consequences for those who receive Botox is that there is a reduction in their ability to read the emotions of those around them. Because Botox essentially paralyzes the muscles of the face, it impairs a person's ability to naturally express emotions via the face, dampening their ability to sense emotions and develop strong connections with those around them. There is a lot going on beyond the conscious mind!

EMOTIONAL TRAUMA

Emotional trauma is just a part of being human. There is no way around it. A traumatic event can best be thought of as any distressing situation that exceeds your ability to emotionally or energetically cope with it, resulting in an incomplete emotional or energetic processing of the experience. The things we perceive in childhood are a little more subtle, complex, and pervasive than many may think. As infants and young children, we have minimal capacity to handle distress because our nervous systems are still in its very early stages of development. It doesn't take much to overwhelm an eight-month-old. Excessive noise, especially on a regular basis, can be too much for a sensitive infant. And what might be traumatic for a 3-year-old might be completely manageable and forgettable for a 12-year-old.

Emotional trauma causes neural fragmentation and the creation of partial ego states that result in the evolution of a neural architecture of personality disorders and low emotional set point for anxiety and fear. Basically, we create personalities and survival strategies to find safety and security because we can't energetically handle the situation. If a child has an adult nervous system that can assist and make them feel safe, they may fully process the overwhelming experience. If not, they may create alternative strategies to cope, manage, or escape the overwhelm.

Birth Trauma

For a newborn, certain aspects of the birthing process itself may be traumatic. If the child is coming into the world with the perception of an immediate danger due to the delivery, the nervous system may be primed to respond to danger if a future threatening environment is perceived. Keep in mind, it doesn't take much to overwhelm a newborn's system. Research suggests some of the modern birth practices may cause trauma, but it's unclear how significant the long-term effects might be. Some of these potential traumas include: the use of forceps during delivery, lack of oxygen supply to the baby's brain from clamping the cord too soon, smacking the infant to initiate crying, and separating baby from mother immediately after delivery. Some of these circumstances may be required for a safe delivery. The point is not to shame the practices, but rather to recognize that the experiences may contribute to the manifestation of mental, emotional, or physical imbalances later in life that we have an opportunity to process and correct. There is plenty of evidence of mothers experiencing post-traumatic stress disorder (PTSD) from birthing. So it shouldn't be a stretch to suspect trauma can affect the newborn as well.

Developmental Trauma

Childhood developmental trauma is undoubtedly the most recognized and well-studied form of trauma. And for most people there are several layers of developmental trauma that create lasting and sometimes lifelong effects. Once again, the age range from birth to around six years old seems to be absolutely critical in determining who we become in adulthood. During this period is when you form many of your ego-based personality patterns, your social strategies, and you lay down your neurobiological foundation and core epigenetic expression.

Many psychiatrists and psychologists throughout the centuries have examined the childhood developmental stages in great depth. Over the past 150 years, notable figures such as Sigmund Freud, Erik Erikson, and Jean Piaget have created detailed and useful theories to describe the psychosocial progression from infancy into adulthood. They have all provided fantastic ways to think about and map the stages of development. In his book *The 5 Personality Patterns*, author Steven Kessler provides one of the more simple ways to think about the psychosocial stages of development and how these stages integrate with emotional trauma, personality patterns, and the associated energetics. Recall that trauma is simply an experience that overwhelms our capacity to energetically or emotionally cope. As it turns out, when a child perceives danger and lacks the emotional tools or caregiver resources to feel safe, the child will create a psychosocial safety strategy—an ego-based form of protection. And as a child experiences significant or repeated trauma, this strategy may develop into disordered personality patterns that can be utilized in the face of emotional overwhelm in the future. You undoubtedly witness expressions of these in your everyday life. Road rage is a perfect example of one pattern. You may know somebody who is an extreme rule follower and is always highly organized. Or you may know somebody who just kind of zones out, shuts down, or mentally disappears in an overwhelming situation. There are many ways these general patterns show up, and they are used in times of emotional or energetic overwhelm.

At each stage, the child gains an ever-increasing sense of independence. First, the child is dependent on the mother in particular, then starts recognizing the self around 18 months old. The child pushes boundaries and starts to explore the world independently. Then the child gains the confidence to stand on his own and develop the self. In this process, the child develops his ego identity and figures out how to operate safely in this world. If the child perceives a safe and secure base in the primary caregivers, he can feel confident to explore the world, make mistakes, and return to safety. If the child does not perceive the necessary connection, safety, and security at each stage of development, this can create not only a personality pattern, but a biological pattern of expression that manifests as an increased fear-based, fight-or-flight response. Until we address the perceived lack of connection, safety, and security in early childhood development, the potential for an elevated fight-or-flight nervous system response exists. The chronic sympathetic overdrive will, over time, contribute to a greater incidence of health issues and disease throughout life.

In my experience, we all experience situations in each stage of childhood development that cause us to create a variety of strategies to navigate the world. Each of us will, however, have one or two dominant strategies that we tend to rely on in most situations.

Adult-Onset Trauma

Of course the potential for introducing trauma doesn't end after childhood. Emotional trauma can be the result of a single, extraordinarily stressful event that dismantles your sense of security and creates a significant sense of fear, or from ongoing stress that engrains a sense of fear or anxiety over time. Common triggers of emotional trauma in adulthood include divorce, severe financial issues, abuse, accidental injury, war, and death of a loved one. While it is uncommon to directly experience a terrorist attack, mass shooting, or natural disasters, the constant barrage of images on television and online can create a chronic trauma-based fear response over time. These common adulthood occurrences reinforce the heightened nervous system response and physiological cascade as a result of being in a fearful or threatened state.

— *Emotional Symptoms:* Shock, denial, disappointment, worry, fear, anger, frustration, sadness, guilt, shame, self-critical, lonely, hopeless, numb, and apathetic, among others

— *Biological Symptoms:* Chronic inflammation, autoimmune conditions, back pain, insomnia, fatigue, elevated blood pressure, hormonal imbalance, skin conditions, diabetes, joint pain, poor digestion, IBS, constipation, diarrhea, leaky gut, and hair loss, among others

Inherited, or Generational, Trauma

One of the more mysterious forms of emotional trauma is that which gets passed down from one generation to the next. In a study from 2013, researchers taught male mice to fear the scent of cherry blossoms by shocking their feet whenever they would introduce the smell. They then bred the males with females who had never been exposed to the smell. The resulting offspring were raised to adulthood having also never been exposed to the scent of cherry blossom. And despite this, when introduced to the scent for the first time, the offspring became anxious and fearful. What's even more amazing is that when the offspring were then bred, the scent of cherry blossom caused anxiety and fear in the next generation as well. Because one generation experiences associative trauma, the effects are still seen two generations later. Some researchers speculate that the noticeable effects of emotional trauma can be observed for seven generations or more.

On the surface, inherited trauma seems a little implausible. But as the science of epigenetics continues to unfold, it begins to make a lot of sense. As a survival mechanism, information about the environment is extremely beneficial to pass on to offspring. This epigenetic adaptation becomes critical for survival in a changing environment. For the mice, the survival adaptation resulted in the offspring being born with an increase in cherry-blossom-detecting neurons and brain space devoted to recognizing cherry blossom, creating a heightened sensitivity to the threat. As the researchers investigated further, they noticed altered DNA methylation activity in the offspring, which alters genetic expression, indicating at least part of the epigenetic mechanism that allows for the transfer of information across generations. In similar studies of human subjects, researchers have demonstrated that the children of Holocaust survivors are more prone to anxiety, depression, and PTSD. Similar to the mouse studies, researchers found an alteration in methylation activity of a stress-related gene, known as FKBP5, in both Holocaust survivors and their children.

Rupert Sheldrake's work on morphic fields, and particularly morphic resonance, provides another potential mechanism through which trauma and environmentally informed conditions might be passed down from one generation to the next. "Through morphic resonance, the patterns of activity in self-organizing systems are influenced by similar patterns in the past, giving each species and each kind of self-organizing system a collective memory," he wrote. Morphic resonance is a thread of connection across time from the past to present. And perhaps the information generated through morphic resonance is simply captured and materialized through epigenetic expression. Unfortunately, because morphic resonance is nonmaterial, science currently has no way to prove or disprove this potential. But this possibility is certainly interesting to consider.

Despite lack of detailed understanding, it is clear that we inherit trauma from our parents and grandparents in such a way that certain aspects of our biology are more attuned and predestined to express in a more dramatic fashion because our ancestors developed a survival adaptation to a given threat. The many possible mechanisms that produce the phenomena of inherited trauma include morphic resonance, epigenetic adaptation, or still some yet undiscovered means by which information gets passed directly through the tissues or the entire system as a whole.

UNDERSTANDING YOUR ATTACHMENT STYLE

In the past few decades, there have been significant efforts made to understand what makes people happy. Countries such as Costa Rica and Bhutan consistently rank at the top of the list of happiest countries on Earth. While there are many factors at play, there are universal contributors that have been identified. Harvard's decades-long research on happiness has shed tremendous light on this subject and, as it turns out, happiness is heavily influenced by personal relationships.

What has been discovered over the past decade is that human connection is fundamental for both happiness, overall health, and, not surprisingly, longevity. For some, human connection is easy. It comes so naturally. For others, establishing authentic human connection can be one of the most terrifying and difficult experiences life has to offer. There are plenty of individuals at each end of the spectrum, but most people in the modern world fall in the middle somewhere.

When it comes to deep connection with a partner and healthy regulation of emotional states in relationships, many individuals run into challenges because of maladaptive attachment styles expressed by them or others. Understanding your own attachment style is very helpful for making relationships work. And developing a more *secure* attachment style is needed for cultivating the deep connections and balanced neurobiology that lead to such profound health effects.

There are three primary attachment styles people use in their most intimate relationships. These have been termed *secure, avoidant,* and *anxious.*

— *Secure:* This attachment style is just as it sounds. These individuals grow up having confidence in the relationship dynamic, and any fear of getting hurt is not significant enough for them to subconsciously create challenges that undermine the desire for deep connection.

— *Avoidant:* This attachment style is the stereotypical role of the male lead in a romantic comedy flick. As the girl shows interest in him, he gets excited about the relationship. Everything goes well for a while until she starts really falling for him. He then freaks out because the relationship is getting real. The more she presses the relationship, the more he backs away and creates distance because his experience has taught him that if he is vulnerable enough to love her deeply, it will lead to severe emotional pain when she leaves him. So he protects against the potential hurt by only letting her get so close. Because individuals with this attachment style have a hard time trusting, they respond well to a slow and steady relationship pace without getting smothered.

— *Anxious:* This attachment style is the stereotypical role of the female lead in a romantic comedy flick. As the guy shows interest in her, she gets excited about the relationship. Everything goes well for a while until she feels like he might not be into her as much as she is into him. Fearing the relationship will stall out, she puts on the full court press, expressing how much she loves him. She also gets very suspicious that he might be talking to other women, so she noses through his phone and Instagram profile. Experience has taught her that love can leave her, so she does everything she can to hang on to it without realizing she's contributing to the destruction. Without a constant reaffirmation of the relationship, individuals with this attachment style tend to fear something is wrong and believe the relationship needs to be fixed or improved.

— *Anxious + Avoidant:* A small percentage of the population will actually rely heavily on both strategies in relationships depending on the situation and their partner's attachment style.

It may not surprise you that our attachment styles primarily form in childhood through relationships with our primary caregivers. The first six years of life prove critical in this regard. This is when children test out reciprocal relationships and learn how to best get their needs met through interactive behavior with others.

A *secure* attachment style develops if children perceive their primary caregivers to be consistently nearby and responsive to their needs, which they express through early methods of communication such as crying, grasping, or smiling. (Later methods include bargaining, negotiation, and compromising.) If a young child perceives her caregivers to be nearby but their responsiveness to her needs is inconsistent, she may use clinging and protesting strategies in an attempt to draw them in. If the child finds this strategy to be successful on a regular basis, then the *anxious* pattern is likely to develop as a successful method to get her needs met. On the other hand, if a child perceives that his primary caregivers are not consistently nearby, or they are nearby but very unresponsive, he may shut down emotionally because he perceives that his needs won't get met. As such, an *avoidant* strategy may develop in order to protect him from getting emotionally hurt.

According to Peter Cummings, the originator of the Adult Attachment Repair Model (AARM), "Attachment trauma is a disorder of ego state functioning. Ego states are charged with the regulation of emotional balance through the biological workings of the central nervous system." This fragmentation of ego states may keep an individual emotionally "stuck," preventing developmental growth toward an integrated, adult ego state capable of healthy emotional modulation.

Internal Working Models

Alongside the development of attachment styles, children also develop an internal working model (IWM) in toddlerhood and beyond in order to navigate social relationships. A child's IWM is an amalgamation of thoughts, emotions, expectations, beliefs, and behaviors generated from early relationship experiences with primary caregivers. There is so much complexity and nuance in the relationship between a child and her primary caregivers. One of the more subtle aspects of relationships that we, as children, pick up on is the quality of emotional and energetic communication. Beyond words and actions, if a child perceives any range of misattuned emotions such as harshness, dismissiveness, humiliation, or anxiety, they will inform her beliefs, meaning, emotions, and thoughts about herself and the world.

Based on early perceptions, children will establish the primary caregivers as caring or hurtful and trustworthy or not. They will begin to think of themselves as good or bad and lovable or unlovable. And they also start to determine if the world is a safe or dangerous place based on perceptions of their experience. Ultimately these perceptions guide the child's level of self-worth and self-acceptance. And because these are subconscious beliefs, they often result in automatic programs that consistently run in the background, influencing thoughts, emotions, and relationship interactions, as well as neurobiology and overall epigenetic expression. Each individual's IWM is applied to relationships with both self and others and continues to develop and evolve through adulthood.

PROCESSING STUCK EMOTION AND REPAIRING RUPTURES

It might be worth stating the obvious at this point—we were all children once. And we all continue to suffer from some level of trauma, attachment disorder, misattunements, ruptures of connection, conditioned beliefs, and maladaptive subconscious programming. While our caregivers certainly played a role in this process, the suffering is created by our own perceptions. A vast majority of caregivers are exceptionally loving and do everything they can for their children. Yet trauma and ruptures in connection still occur, no matter how amazing the caregivers were. It is an impossible task for a caregiver to raise an unblemished child.

There is a very wide spectrum of experiences, perceptions, and conditioning that each of us has carried into adulthood. While it is often tempting to look for the *best* method to heal trauma, in my experience, it can be extremely beneficial to view the many therapeutic methods as a buffet. There may be specific methods or practitioners that really call out to you, great—lean into them! The invitation is to also sample the therapeutic menu, because each method and practitioner may have a different "medicine" for you. There are so many pieces to your unique puzzle. Depending on which experiences are still unprocessed or unworked, the most effective way forward for you might be to utilize a handful of methods, as each method has its strengths. Let your intuition guide you and trust that your body knows *exactly* what to do!

Adult Attachment Repair Model

AARM is a method of improving disorganized attachment styles and fragmented ego states by retraining the neurobiological pathways through corrective somatic experience. This method incorporates a right-brain therapeutic approach of interacting, sensing, and feeling in order to address maladaptive behaviors and negative thought patterns stemming from early parent-child interactions. It is difficult to encapsulate the profundity of this method, as the mechanisms of action are quite simple, but the practitioner's execution is exquisitely deep and nuanced.

Hypnotherapy

While it does require finding a quality practitioner, hypnotherapy can be an extremely effective way to get to the subconscious stories that are running in the background. By increasing slow-wave brain activity, "side-stepping" aspects of the conscious mind, and reprogramming the subconscious thoughts, feelings, and beliefs through hypnotherapy, tremendous resolution can be achieved in relatively short order.

Eye Movement Desensitization and Reprocessing (EMDR)

EMDR is a method used to address both isolated traumatic events and prolonged or repeated traumatic experiences. EMDR is frequently applied in cases of PTSD to reduce sensitivity to distressing memories related to the traumatic event. The process utilizes rhythmic, side-to-side sensory inputs generated by either visual, auditory, or tactile stimuli in conjunction with cognitive recall of the distressing event in an effort to stabilize adaptive beliefs and emotions around traumatic experiences.

EMDR is essentially working to remove the blocks preventing the complete neurobiological and emotional processing of painful events. There are a number of scientific studies demonstrating the effectiveness of EMDR at resolving PTSD and other responses to trauma.

Indigenous Sacred Plant Medicines

Ceremonial use of psychoactive plants such as ayahuasca, iboga, San Pedro cactus, and psilocybin mushrooms in the presence of a highly qualified practitioner or vetted indigenous healer has proven to be remarkably effective at releasing stored emotional traumas, rebalancing the autonomic nervous system, and helping the individual to find new perspective and meaning. While completely safe for most people, it should be avoided by those with heart conditions, blood pressure issues, or liver or kidney dysfunctions, as well as those who have certain psychiatric conditions.

According to the wisdom of indigenous healers and my own personal experience, the role of the facilitator plays a significant role in the process not only from a safety perspective but also in terms of therapeutic effectiveness. Indigenous cultures regard these plants and their use as sacred. While generally regarded as safe, recreationally or carelessly utilizing these natural compounds can sometimes create a more difficult psychological or emotional process in the long-term, so it is best to work with these plants only if you feel called to do so. It is also recommended that you work with these in the presence of an experienced practitioner and in an environment in which you feel completely safe.

While it shouldn't be expected that a single experience will resolve everything in an instant, the experiences can be quite profound and may result in miraculous resolution of mental, emotional, and physical illness. For many individuals, however, it can be beneficial to work with these plants many, many times, resulting in progressive improvement and a deepening of the experience. For reference, many indigenous ayahuasca practitioners drink and serve ayahuasca many thousands of times over the course of their lives.

Rolfing and Block Therapy

Rolfing is a form of bodywork that specifically targets the connective tissue throughout the body, known as fascia, in order to create better energy flow. It removes energetic blockages in the body, increases flow, and facilitates greater structural balance and systemic coordination, by which the stored energy from emotional trauma can be freed and processed. By stimulating the intrafascial sensory neurons, Rolfing reduces the tension held in the muscles and fascia.

Block Therapy is a self-practice that also targets the fascial networks. By strategically lying on a hard bamboo block in a variety of ways and using focused diaphragmatic breathing, you can methodically break apart fascial adhesions and improve the delivery of nitric oxide, oxygen, blood, and life-force energy to all your cells and tissues. This unwinds the fascia, opens up the subtle energetic channels and cellular architecture, and allows for greater processing of trapped energy and emotion held in the body.

Holotropic Breath Work

Many forms of breath work can be effective at balancing the autonomic nervous system, increasing parasympathetic tone, and providing relief from emotionally challenging experiences. Holotropic appears to be one of the most effective approaches for actually releasing trauma stored in the subconscious (and body tissues) through the intense circular breathing style over the course of 30 to 60 minutes. This can be done on your own, but it may be more effective in a class setting with an instructor guiding the process.

Holotropic breath work helps to bring overwhelming experiences, thoughts, emotions, and memories from the subconscious to the conscious, resulting in a cathartic expression—a release and processing of emotion that usually involves the body. It is not uncommon to shake, cry, laugh, experience intense emotion, have an out-of-body experience, or go into a deep, trance-like state. According to Zen master Thich Nhat Hanh, "Breath is the bridge which connects life to consciousness, which unites your body to your thoughts. Whenever your mind becomes scattered, use your breath as the means to take hold of your mind again." When it comes to conscious regulation of the body, the breath holds the top spot!

Forgiveness Work

There's a popular saying that resentment is like drinking poison in the hopes that your enemies die. There is real wisdom in this proverb. Through the process of forgiveness, we can find tremendous therapeutic value.

Research indicates that most individuals resist forgiving their perpetrators because holding on to the anger and resentment makes them feel powerful. Real forgiveness work is a lot more challenging than most recognize. In many circumstances, full forgiveness is achieved through methodical and consistent practice. Rarely is it achieved in a single fell swoop.

Ho'oponopono is an ancient forgiveness *practice* that is simple and effective if used with intention, dedication, and regularity. As Dr. Ihaleakala Hew Len outlines, Ho'oponopono is about taking 100 percent responsibility for anything you are aware of without feeling guilt or shame. The process involves repeating four phrases:

1. I love you.
2. Please forgive me.
3. I am sorry.
4. Thank you.

Through this simple practice, you can initiate self-transformation by cleansing yourself of the trapped subconscious emotions related to a person, place, or event. Used like a mantra, it is simply a process of letting go without intellectualizing or judging anything.

Another method, espoused by psychotherapist and Ayurvedic practitioner Dr. Keesha Ewers, involves listing the "negative" character traits of the person who has wronged you. After you list the many traits that are associated with the person who offended you, you then recognize how you exhibit those same traits in your interpersonal relationships. Through this process, you can begin to consciously recognize that the other person is no different than you—that we are all "guilty" of wronging others. As such, the process of forgiving the "other" and forgiving yourself is one and the same. Paradoxically, the process of forgiving others is really about forgiving yourself. And therein lies the ultimate medicine.

Family Constellation Therapy

This is a powerful therapeutic tool to help process unresolved trauma specifically related to family relationship dynamics and complex family entanglements. The process reveals hidden or subconscious social dynamics in your family relationships in order to bring conscious awareness to remove the psychosocial and emotional barriers to healthy connection. This can also act as an effective method to address transgenerational patterns of emotional and energetic entanglements.

The subconscious mind has immense implications on health and longevity. If the subconscious is filled with the perception of fear, loneliness, self-criticism, shame, guilt, disappointment, anger, sadness, and the like, the autonomic nervous system will exhibit an exaggerated baseline, sympathetic fight-or-flight expression. When the body is dedicating energy and genetic expression to survival processes, it has little energy to dedicate to repair and rejuvenation. Any inherited traumas can also affect the development of biological expression in a child. If, due to emotional traumas and subconscious beliefs, a child's nervous system dedicates additional energy to a sympathetic, fight-or-flight expression, the gut ecosystem, brain, immune system, and overall epigenetic expression suffers into adulthood as a consequence. Ultimately, this can result in a reduced capacity to harmonize with the environment, creating more cellular damage, greater propensity for disease, and acceleration of the aging process.

Chapter 9

PRACTICE MINDFULNESS

---

*As far as we can discern, the sole purpose of human existence is to
kindle a light in the darkness of mere being.*

— CARL JUNG

It was our fourth day on the island of Ikaria, Greece, and we
were settling into the flow of the quiet and serene village life on the
north side of the island. Long trips through the winding mountain passes rewarded us with picturesque views of the neighboring
islands and cyaneous Agean Sea. As we arrived in the lively port
town of Agios Kirikos, bustling with midsummer tourist activity,
the car just ahead of ours slowly came to a stop next to the car in
the oncoming lane, blocking both sides of the small road. Both
drivers rolled down their windows and began chatting. Patiently,
we waited for them to finish saying their hellos. From our van-
tage point, the conversation appeared friendly and jovial, with the
occasional head nod and a myriad of hand gestures. After a couple
minutes passed, we began to get a little confused. Did they not see
that we were stuck behind them? Without our Greek translator in
tow, there was little we could communicate. But nobody else was
honking their horn, so we waited, curiously. Perhaps one of them
has car trouble, we thought. Then at the five-minute mark, we
couldn't help but laugh as they continued to chat, windows down,

blocking the road—with no other drivers creating a fuss. It was clear to us at that point that this is just how it is in Ikaria. What's more important than connecting with a friend when you see one? And every other driver seemed to agree as they patiently waited. It set us straight as we realized the deep truth these locals embodied.

You might be able to get away with this in the smallest of U.S. towns. But had this kind of thing happened anywhere else in the United States, neighboring drivers would have likely created a scene—and I can't say I wouldn't be doing the same. In Ikaria, the only "horns" were those atop the heads of goats grazing in nearby fields. Nobody was in a rush, it seemed.

The values held by the locals were completely skewed from what I grew up knowing. Sure, we talk about the importance of slowing down, reducing stress, having patience, and the benefits of social interaction, but it isn't embodied and exhibited like we saw in Ikaria and the other longevity cultures we visited. I recall Orestis Portelos of Ikaria saying, "There has always been something special about our island, because people never go over the edge. There is compassion, solidarity, and all these things that are able to connect people in order to avoid fights between each other." This was quite the contrast to the narrower societal focus on our own needs and personal desires that I was used to: My time is more important than yours. I was here first. You owe me this. You did not put in your fair share. You are invading my space.

Spending time with the elders in their hometowns was one of the greatest gifts I've been given. These cultures acted as a beautiful mirror for me to acutely examine the conditioning of my own thoughts and beliefs, and how I have reflexively moved through life. It was interesting to consider where my unconscious thoughts and behaviors originated. These self-centered, impatient, and critical values weren't explicitly taught to me by my parents. In fact, quite the opposite. I don't recall any schoolteacher, coach, or mentor ever consciously instilling these values in me either. Rather they seem to be immature aspects from a childhood identity that I hadn't yet grown out of and that were socially conditioned and culturally reinforced.

Because I was not used to seeing people in public behave in such a manner, it caught my attention. It was such a stark contrast to what I was used to seeing that it, in one instant, had me examining an entire subset of values, thoughts, and beliefs I had about community, connection, and the pace of society. It wasn't that I woke up to how society *should* behave. Rather, I didn't even conceive that it was possible for society to behave in such a fashion.

The funny thing about our conditioned beliefs and ideas is that, at first glance, it can seem impossible to recognize, accept, and truly embody a different way of being. It's as if we are missing a part of the map or the instruction book. And once you have the missing pieces, it all seems so simple, so obvious. And the first part of the process is bringing awareness to the misalignments and limited perspectives. My intent for this chapter is to shine a light on some of these and offer a few tools to help you open up to a more expanded, integrated, and coherent reality that invites in greater health and well-being.

DISCONNECTION

As industry and technology boomed in the West over the past 200 years, advancements in transportation and communication created larger, more densely populated cities. Paradoxically, as we began to live closer together and communication became easier, meaningful interaction declined and authentic connection suffered. Simultaneously, urban sprawl and increased economic independence led to greater separation from the extended family and fostered isolation from a once-familiar community. In the process, collective values were supplanted, while community-entrenched morals and virtues slowly gave way to individual pleasure, comfort, and entertainment.

By the late 20th century, technological advancement and economic prosperity provided such profound safety and security, many no longer required close interaction with the environment or community as a means of survival. Along with disengaging from the environment and each other, we began losing touch with our sense of responsibility and meaning in the world. Even now, as greater convenience and comfort seeps into every aspect of our lives, we often struggle to sit still, silence our thoughts, and just be.

One of the most effective ways to foster greater collective action is through social institutions. Historically, all over the world, social institutions are fundamental to the collective structure—they typically include marriage, extended family, religious groups, nongovernmental civic organizations, and the like. Prior to industrialization, societies were more reliant on the extended family unit to provide safety and security for all. Larger families helped ensure there would be enough hands to work the fields, take care of the household, and help look after the young children and elderly. With the Industrial Revolution and greater economic growth, more and more children started going to school. As the father often worked away from home to generate income necessary to afford modern conveniences, the mother often stayed home to do the busy job of tending to the household and children. Then, with the progress of women's rights, more women began entering the workforce, gaining financial independence of their own. Then as both men and women garnered an opportunity to pursue their passions and earn an income independently, the dynamic of the family unit shifted. Divorce became more common and parents weren't spending as much time together with their children. Grandparents no longer had to rely on the extended family for care because they developed the financial means to pay for professional support and care.

What's interesting to note is that the progress that's been made in terms of women's rights, reducing the poverty rate, and an increase in children going to school are inherently beneficial to health and longevity. Along the way, however, we seem to have lost some of the social structures that foster connection, support, responsibility, and purpose. Formal and informal social institutions at the local level create a sense of unity and shared common goal. Without the smaller group collectives intact, it becomes much more difficult for the individual to develop a connection to large collective groups composed of thousands. When the elders were young, competition was in balance with collective action. The whole was not superseded by the individual. And small group collectives were highly valued because they provided greater safety, security, and well-being for the individual and their neighbor.

THE TIES THAT BIND

So many of us have increasingly felt it. With the explosion of social media and its influence on society, communication has dramatically increased while personal relationships have suffered. In response to the feeling that something is missing, many are intentionally seeking out like-minded individuals in an attempt to restore "community."

The need for community has become a central talking point among many experts in the fields of public health and social science. Humans are social creatures, and we depend on interaction with others. There's an entire research field of social genomics dedicated to learning more about the role social behavior plays in epigenetic expression. I want to point to the idea that there is more that we are seeking and needing beyond the generic concept of community. Most dictionaries define *community* as a group of people with shared attitudes, interests, or characteristics. So while community *could* be beneficial, it is also quite possible to be part of a community and still feel completely isolated and unsupported.

Connection, safety, support, and belonging are the essence or glue that holds community together and gives it strength. To feel like you belong somewhere or with somebody is a feeling that carries with it acceptance and love for who you are. It's like feeling at home. So perhaps it isn't community, but rather it is deep connection, safety, support, and acceptance that many of us in the modern world are so badly craving.

For the elders, it was not uncommon to grow up with 5 to 10 siblings, maybe more. Grandparents often helped raise the grandchildren, and each new generation would eventually help take care of the older generations as they aged. It was much less common for young people to move away and find a new home. This drove strong, lifelong family connections and profound moral responsibility for the elders throughout their life. The strong social fabric was born and sustained out of necessity, and greater well-being was supplied through cooperation within families and between neighbors. Resources were often shared in an egalitarian manner, making sure to support those in desperate need of assistance.

In Okinawa, 85-year-old businessman Fuji Sasaki described an old tradition known as a *moai* that he participated in with a dozen other men and women in town. Each month, they'd meet up, and each contributed money into a collective fund. When somebody in the group, or even one of their family members, needed any social or financial support in a time of hardship, they would use the collective funds to offer assistance. These *moai* groups regularly meet for decades in support of one another. The *moai* serves as insurance for each of the members, providing a social and financial safety net that is independent of any formal legal entity.

Georgios Stenos of Ikaria told stories of a similar concept they call *allaksia*, which is a system of mutual aid. A couple members of the village might come help Georgios with a large project he was working on. Later, when the others requested assistance, he would offer his services to help them complete a needed task. They would act as laborers for one another in a bartering fashion, recognizing that if they worked together, they could accomplish a great deal more. The reason these types of exchanges work is because they have established connections with one another. They feel a sense of commitment and moral obligation to assist and support one another because they have built a relationship of mutual aid, care, and support. They help each other for the betterment of the community and ultimately, themselves. The healthier the community, the healthier the individual, and vice versa.

This type of egalitarian societal structure is difficult for large cities with dense populations. The more people there are, the harder it becomes to pool and share resources because the connection to the whole and sense of moral obligation is so easily diffused in large populations. But if small, local groups reengage one another, there is a tremendous opportunity to enhance connection, provide support, and increase the sense of security and well-being. This not only translates to improved mood and emotional states, this translates to biology and can dramatically improve physical health.

There is now a large body of scientific research detailing the cellular mechanisms and epigenetic changes that occur as a result of social influences. A chronic lack of connection has been shown to down-regulate genes related to protective immune function while up-regulating proinflammatory genes. When social connection is lacking, the body responds with an increased stress response in preparation for conditions of threat. And if your nervous system and physiology are conditioned to easily tip into fight or flight, your ability to repair and regenerate is diminished while the likelihood of nearly all chronic inflammatory conditions increases. It should be of little surprise that mood conditions such as depression, anxiety, and addiction are highly influenced by social influences and lack of connection.

Increasing social connection and safety have very meaningful impacts on physiology, mood, and cellular health. This is just one more example of how invisible environmental energies—in this case, connection—can influence beliefs, thoughts, and emotions that control biological expression in profound ways. And this is precisely what the ongoing Harvard Happiness Study, which began in 1938, suggests. They found close relationships were the primary predictor of happiness over the course of their test subjects' lives. These ties that bind appear to be more influential on health and happiness than inherited genes, money, and social status. The 80-plus-year longitudinal study revealed that loneliness is actually more harmful to your health than smoking or alcoholism. Researchers also found that those with strong social support were able to better deal with life's stresses, maintaining greater physical, mental, and emotional health over time.

While researchers are beginning to see the importance of connection on biological function, there seems to be a slight disconnect when it comes to understanding how to actually create connection. For some, connection can seem quite natural. And yet many others have a difficult time developing deep connections that provide enough security and support to influence our body systems in a harmonious way. Establishing connection requires a certain level of safety and trust. While the desire and need for connection is inborn, the ability to connect is something that we learn to establish. And as mentioned in the previous chapter, connection is first influenced by our attachment styles and personality patterns that develop in relation to our primary caregivers in the first six years of life or so.

The multitude of influences continue through various developmental stages, further affecting our ability to socially connect. From childhood into young adulthood, we learn to navigate relationships with peers and authority figures. And as bizarre as it may sound, connection can actually feel dangerous and disconcerting in adulthood. If we never established secure connection and attachment in childhood, we then crave connection as adults. But because we couldn't count on it as children, even just getting a hint of it can trigger the pain of it disappearing or becoming unavailable. So oftentimes, we find it very difficult to actually open up and relax into real connection. Our fight-or-flight sympathetic nervous system can activate as if connection itself is a threat. What may be required is a certain level of nervous system modulation, reprogramming, and co-regulation with another in order to begin to trust and feel safe in the body when connection is offered. For some, the ruptures in childhood were so deep and significant, it can take months or years of reprogramming the nervous system with a trained professional. In my experience, Adult Attachment Repair Model, mentioned in the previous chapter, offers one of the most powerful solutions to this type of dysregulated pattern.

This is why safe and secure relationship dynamics in the immediate and extended family play a significant role in fostering a local community that has the capacity to develop rich social connection, provide support, and offer a social security that fosters health over disease. This is what seemed to be cultivated when the elders were young and throughout their lives. And, from what I could see, it still exists in the small villages today.

There are also broader aspects of connection that don't involve another person. Because almost all human relationships are perceived as conditional instead of unconditional, we learn that opening up to connection involves risk of getting hurt. But if you perceived the relationship as unconditional and without risk of getting hurt, it would feel much easier and safer to connect. Perhaps this is one reason most people love animals so much. Human-to-animal connection has been shown by research to deliver very similar results as human-to-human connection. Children who read to animals have shown improved social skills, increased cooperation, fewer behavior problems, and a greater desire to volunteer. And in children without siblings, pet ownership helps them develop greater empathy and better self-esteem. It shouldn't be surprising that researchers are uncovering similar biological mechanisms as those found in human-human connection. Interacting with animals increases feelings of social support and a reduced feeling of isolation, which results in a down regulation of fight-or-flight sympathetic nervous system activity. Consequently, a reduction of cortisol levels has been found along with reduced blood pressure and cholesterol. In the elderly, pet ownership has been shown to improve their ability to perform everyday physical activities such as climbing stairs, preparing meals, and bathing.

There are other ways humans can develop connection as well. Religious and nonreligious people alike are constantly fostering a connection with their idea of the creator or an aspect of life that is larger than their ego-based personality. According to research, this also improves mental, emotional, and physical health. Students of Buddhism and similar forms of spiritual practice are, in a way, developing a connection with deeper aspects of themselves and their true nature—leading to the embodied realization that they are never disconnected from anything.

Based on the science of social genomics, connection is proving to be a fundamental need by all humans. And this can come in many forms—connection with other people, with animals, the creator, nature, and ourselves. Opening up to any or all of these connections is a very worthwhile endeavor. The more connection we feel, the more coherent our biological expression and sense of well-being.

DEEPER MEANING

James Hollis, author of *Finding Meaning in the Second Half of Life*, suggests that more people suffer from a disconnect of meaning than from any other source of injury.

Imagine placing yourself in the shoes of an 18-year-old Michelino Scudu. You're working as a shepherd and living in the little commune of Villagrande Strisaili in the mountains of Sardinia. It is summer in the year 1935. You have no running water or electricity, so you source your water from streams and mountain springs as you walk your sheep 40 miles. Fortunately, this clean mountain water is some of the best water you'll find in Sardinia. Unfortunately, the spring and summer have been remarkably warm and you're in the midst of a dry spell. If you don't get adequate water to your large family garden soon, you'll lose the harvest and winter could be challenging. Now compare this to our life today. Who likely places greater value and meaning in the ability to source water?

I asked Michelino what makes living in the mountains of Sardinia so good for human health. Here's how he responded: "Because there are lots of forests and natural springs with healthy water. Water is very important for the well-being. If it's good, it fulfills you. And here the water is very good. It's very important for your health. Different than the water you find in the Campidano area. This comes directly from the mountains. I worked a lot in the Gennargentu Mountains, where every 20 meters you can find a spring. I used to eat *casu axedu*, or goat meat, and drink that water, the main elixir for long life. Water is a very important element when it comes to longevity."

Your experiences of the reality in which you live generate subtle or not-so-subtle feelings. From these feelings a perception is generated, be it clear or distorted, accurate or inaccurate in the truest sense. From the perception of the feeling, meaning is then created, which then influences behavior and experience. Until we bring conscious awareness to this cyclical process, most of it is happening on the subconscious level based on our conditioning.

Experience → Feeling → Perception → Meaning → Behavior
→ Experience → Feeling, etc.

As I began to understand the circumstances and lifestyles of the elders when they were younger, it was quite interesting to consider what was meaningful to them and compare that with what is meaningful for people living in the industrialized world. For example, many in the United States today assign a great deal of meaning to financial security and wealth. We often define success by our material possessions, social status, degrees, and accomplishments. There is a great deal of meaning in things like money, entertainment, technology, and fashion because the experiences and perceptions generated in the United States are very centered around these things. Or we might assign a great deal of meaning to things like the Super Bowl, social media activity, or which brand of shoes to buy. While none of this is inherently wrong or bad, it also seems that much of it fails to contribute much to our health and well-being. In contrast, more of the elders' experiences centered around life-affirming principles—sourcing good water, tending to their gardens, supporting others in the community, and religious or spiritual practices. These experiences led to feelings and perceptions that created meaning which was centered around survival, the good of the community, and God.

So many of the things we take for granted in the modern world weren't even a part of the elders' reality when they were young.

Things such as electricity, central heating, refrigeration, Internet, automobiles, emergency rooms, and antibiotics. So many of us even take our meals for granted, often eating alone in front of a screen. Not only did the elders of Okinawa typically eat together, but they have a practice of gratitude before they eat. They say *Itadakimasu,* which is loosely translated as, "I receive the life of this food to benefit my own life. Thank you for this meal." The deeper meaning is associated with having gratitude for every living being that is responsible for the meal—from the plants, animals, farmer, chef, and so on. There are many layers of meaning embedded in this one little word. Even the four- or five-year-olds would say this before eating.

It became quite apparent that the cultures in which the elders lived actually had a keen sense of awareness around where they placed meaning and that some of it was consciously cultivated in a variety of rituals and practices. And this highlights the opportunity we all have—to get curious about where we are placing meaning in our life and examining if it truly serves our health and well-being and is in alignment with our dream—or if it is keeping us caught in a maladaptive, subconscious, conditioned response.

As you bring greater conscious awareness to the conditioned patterns and where you place meaning, you can then interrupt the subconscious cycle anywhere in the process.

Experience → Feeling → Perception → Meaning → Behavior → Experience → Feeling, etc.

In other words, you can reprogram this process by bringing it from the subconscious to the conscious. The two easiest ways to consciously do this are to:

1. Modify your behavior, which will help change the experience, feeling, perception, and meaning. You can create rituals or practices that align with principles that are important to you.

2. Choose where you want to place meaning, and this will help you figure out how to modify your behavior to achieve this.

It may take some consideration to determine how to best implement this into your life. But this is a practice that, over time, will create new neural circuits and programs that improve health and well-being.

Responsibility

For the elders, one of the things that gave them meaning was a heavy load of responsibility. When I asked Vitalio Melis of Sardinia what he thinks contributed to his long and healthy life, he said, "At fourteen, I started to work with my father in the countryside, farming and everything else. It was a hard life of sacrifice and effort. But I did it with love, and I was always happy. I was always healthy, thank God. Even now, I don't take any medicine. I am 91 and so the age is there. And even this morning, I was in the vegetable garden to get beans, lettuce, and so on."

They had to look after their land, the food they grew, their livestock, family, greater community, and their health. They didn't have the luxury of having doctors and hospitals that could deliver acute medical care if something went wrong. And they certainly didn't have grocery stores in case food was running low. The elders had a lot less room for error with everything they did, which forced responsibility and imbued meaning into their everyday lives. The Japanese term *ikigai* is loosely translated as "a reason for being." The word *iki* translates to "life" and *gai* means "value" or "worth." So it really is about that thing that gives your life value. And the elders I spoke with in Okinawa told me they defined it as "what I'm doing is meaningful and I'm happy that I'm doing it."

Meaning in the Mundane

One of the things I took notice of was how many of the elders found meaning in the mundane. It was as if they consciously chose to infuse meaning in the simplest of things to remind them of what's important in life—even the rising of the morning sun. The Okinawans often say the phrase *nuchi gusui yasa* to describe an experience that's "good for the soul." It could be as simple as laughing together or sharing a meal with friends, or dancing, yet they were keenly aware of the subtle aspects of life that really impacted their well-being. Meaning was embedded in so much of the Okinawan way of life that it was a bit challenging for a Westerner like me to keep up. While a bit foreign to me, their customs always seemed to have a life-affirming quality, which I found quite beautiful. It was then that I realized that we have the opportunity to generate and infuse meaning into any aspect of our lives. As my indigenous Peruvian friend Puma says, "Jason, I am always in ceremony." The more life-affirming meaning you can infuse into the small, mundane, and seemingly insignificant tasks, the greater meaning your entire life will hold.

What Is Purpose?

I expected the elders to share how their life was infused with great purpose. Having a purpose in life has been extensively highlighted in previous research and anthropological studies as a critical factor for health and longevity. Surprisingly, I found quite the opposite with the elders—at least not the kind of purpose I was familiar with.

My idea of purpose was associated with status or a specific endeavor that gives meaning to one's life. The elders didn't really think in this way at all. They didn't need to *do* anything specific to give their life meaning or importance. They all seemed to give great importance to life itself and their way of *being*. If anything stood out to me, it was their character and moral compass. They worked hard, supported their loved ones, treated people with respect, and were grateful for whatever they had. If anything, this was their purpose.

Adolfo Melis of Sardinia, the 94-year-old middle of the three Melis brothers, adamantly said, "It's like this: be calm, peaceful, talk to everybody, love everybody. Always have a dialogue, an exchange, but always being calm. And love everybody. And also help others when you can."

At 85, Georgios Stenos thought the main reason people of Ikaria live such long lives was that they treated each other as equals and lived in harmony. He also added, "Nobody was jealous of their neighbor and nobody was exploited." According to the elders I met, they didn't even think about purpose in their life.

I spoke at length with University of Michigan professor and researcher Vic Strecher, who wrote the book *Life on Purpose*. And he defines purposeful as "applying your best self to what matters most." This definition highlights why it is so important to bring awareness to where you are currently placing meaning. Is it on something trivial or is it in alignment with your dream or objective? His definition also highlights the importance of getting clear on your dream or objective, so you can determine what is meaningful for you. Vic's definition perfectly encapsulates the way the elders lived and the way of their cultures in general.

Many of the elders also spoke of balance and moderation. I asked 92-year-old George Stenos of Ikaria what advice he would give to younger generations. He replied, "Professional life should be simple, not in a constant chase for money. A simple moderate life. Neither too wealthy, nor too poor. Neither too much anxiety, nor chasing. Peaceful living."

Ines Pittau of Sardinia, at 103 years old, gave very similar advice for living a long and healthy life when she said, "Live healthy and calmly. And peace. That is important. You go to church, you pray to God that He may send you health. And peace. All of this peace with everyone. That is the main thing, peace." If you didn't catch that, peace was pretty important to Ines. It was amazing how many of the elders stressed this point. Treating others with kindness and compassion was at the top of their lists.

I also found it interesting that none of the elders had ambitions to pursue what we in the West might call a "big life," and instead were plenty content living a quiet life of humility. Professor Vic Strecher told me a story about the many days he spent in a children's hospital when his daughter was sick and required a heart transplant. He took notice of a janitor who, in addition to his regular duties, would visit with and read to the sick kids who weren't regularly visited by parents or loved ones. He and I were both tearing up as he told this story of a man who had clearly found significant meaning beyond his work as a janitor.

REDUCE STIMULATION

As our short flight from Rome touched down on the island of Sardinia, filmmaker John Dahlgren and I couldn't help but notice the dramatic change of pace between the busy city streets of Sardinia's main city of Cagliari and the quaint mountain villages in which the elders lived. After just a three-hour drive north, we arrived in Villagrande to a familiar sight that reminded us of the villages in Guanacaste, Costa Rica, and the island of Ikaria. In every village square, you'll find every public bench occupied by local elders, sitting there enjoying the day without a care in the world. Even as visitors, rushing, with a limited time to get our work done, the slow and peaceful energy of the village had a calming effect on us. Not a single person in the village appeared hurried and, as hard as it might be to imagine, mobile technology was completely absent in public—even among the kids. Not only did they live a calm and stress-free life, but the level of stimulation in Villagrande Strisaili was a fraction of what we experienced in Cagliari and what's typical in most of the modern world. It was interesting to hear from the elders across the world that they didn't have many structured mindfulness practices to help deal with mental or emotional stress. Instead, there was a natural, slow pace embedded into the village cultures of Costa Rica, Sardinia, Ikaria, and Okinawa. The only formal practice that was mentioned was in Okinawa, called *shinrin-yoku*, which translates to "forest bathing." This is the simple practice of immersing yourself in nature and allowing the Nature to work her magic. The precise mechanisms are still being elucidated, but evidence points to the energies, sights, sounds, and smells of nature all working together to activate a parasympathetic (rest and digest) nervous system response. Studies show that even looking at a photo of nature or having plants in the home have a similar effect—lowering cortisol, blood pressure, heart rate, and improving mood.

As engagement with technology continues to have greater influence across humanity and communication becomes ever more instantaneous, the benefits of disconnecting and reducing overall stimulation will likely increase. Finding silence or darkness in a U.S. city today is next to impossible. Phone calls, texts, e-mails, video games, movies, and music now follow us everywhere we go, injected into every aspect of our lives. While this might have sounded like an amazing dream 20 years ago, it has brought with it a lot of complication. In fact, many in the United States are turning to digital detox retreats as a way to escape technology for even a few days of relief. The level of stimulation and fast pace of life in modern, industrial societies is unparalleled in human history.

The constant pings, dings, buzzes, rings, horns, sirens, and flashes are occupying our auditory and visual fields like never before. And because this level of collective stimulation is relatively new to our biology, our brain and nervous system have a limited capacity to adapt. While we've now become accustomed to operating in this environment, on a biological level, we haven't sufficiently adapted in a way that maintains balance and coherence in the system. And when your brain's limbic system is activated by constant noise and things quickly entering your visual field, your biological systems are wired to either fight or flee. Overstimulation activates the sympathetic nervous system and may create a host of mental/emotional conditions, ranging from anxiety and depression to PTSD, ADD, and ADHD. An overactivation of the sympathetic nervous system has even been shown to cause neurogenic inflammation. This inflammatory cascade is caused by sensory input to the brain, but it may occur anywhere in the body. In an effort to reduce inflammation, many people change their diet, add anti-inflammatory supplements, and improve their lifestyle but still get stuck in an inflammatory state. They just don't recognize the importance of reducing stimulation to the brain. When the nervous system is stuck in sympathetic overdrive, you have a decreased ability to adapt to the environment, and thus your capacity for healing is hindered. By slowing things down and minimizing sensory stimulation, you support parasympathetic nervous system activity and facilitate greater healing. There are a number of strategies you can implement to consciously slow things down in a fast-paced world. Here are a few of them.

Engage with Nature

In the modern world, as much as 90 percent or more of waking hours are spent indoors. This ratio was essentially reversed in the elders' societies, just as it was throughout nearly all human history. The more you can engage your senses with nature, the greater benefit you'll realize. Take a walk in the woods, go camping, swim in the ocean, lie in the grass, go for a hike, go skiing. Being active in nature can provide a calming medicine to your nervous system.

Go Inward

There are many ways to go inward and reduce external stimulation. Meditation, breath work, yoga, prayer, qigong, tai chi, and float tanks are just some of the ways to slow things down and focus awareness on the more subtle aspects of the body and mind. Find your preferred methods and incorporate them into your daily routine as much as possible. You don't have to be an expert to start. The simple act of engaging these practices has meaningful effects on your nervous system, physiology, mood, sense of self, and overall well-being.

Ditch the Electronics

Would it surprise you to know that, according to recent research on happiness in teens, any activity that involved a screen correlated with a greater sense of unhappiness? And every activity surveyed that didn't involve a screen, including doing homework, was linked to greater happiness? Have you considered how your life might be different if you changed your relationship with electronic devices?

You can make it a practice to shut off your mobile phone, leave it at home, or set it to airplane mode. Trade the e-reader for real, physical books. Disengage from headphones and earbuds to and give your auditory sense a break from constant stimulation. Take regular, multiday breaks from social media or delete the apps from your phone entirely. The only way to honestly evaluate your relationship with the electronics in your life is to get curious about how they affect your mental and emotional state and radically shift your usage. I invite you to go two days or a week without using your mobile phone at all. Maybe you delete Instagram from your phone. Or perhaps you can experiment with turning the TV off for two weeks straight, or even a month. The idea is to simply observe, without judgment, what emotions, sensations, feelings, and patterns arise as you experiment with things like this so you can create greater levels of awareness around how these electronics are affecting your well-being.

Create

One of the more impactful ways to improve mental, emotional, and physical health is to bring more physical creative expression into your life through dance, art, music, and the like. Art therapy has been successfully used for decades. While creative pursuits aren't absent from modern society, they have been largely replaced by technology. Whether its digital music creation, digital photography and art, or the use of film editing software, these creative pursuits don't deliver the same level of mind-body connection that playing guitar, painting, singing, or dancing can provide. These types of creative expression become especially important as we get older, as they have been shown to protect against cognitive decline and neurodegenerative disorders.

FROM NEGATIVE TO POSITIVE

The amygdala, one of the primitive parts of your brain, is said to use about two-thirds of its capacity to identify danger. And once it does, the perceptions and experiences get immediately stored into your memory for later use—a brilliant system to keep you alive. Interestingly, in the modern world, there are very few life-threating scenarios that most of us experience. Yet this part of the brain still tends to dominate the equation. Scientific research suggest that upward of 75 percent of our thoughts are of the "negative" persuasion, which is known as the negativity bias. For those who experienced a great deal of trauma in childhood or perceived a consistent lack of love, support, and connection, the negativity bias is likely to operate on overdrive.

While it can be extremely beneficial to work with and process underlying traumas and subconscious perceptions, research has shown that some individuals genetically inherit unhappiness. On the plus side, there is also an opportunity to consciously change this neurological pattern such that the default program is to look for and notice the good. Research shows that positivity is primarily guided by thoughts and behaviors. All it takes is consistent practice and you can rewire your brain, increase your baseline positivity level, and make joy your default operating system.

Gratitude Practice

The Okinawan elders we met with practice gratitude every time they sit down for a meal. Gratitude for them was nothing less than the recognition of a positive aspect in their life. This conscious recognition of even simple things in life is a powerful way to positively influence your nervous system and mood. The following is one practice you can implement: At night, write down all the things that you can think of that upset you during the day—as many as you like. When you are finished, safely burn or throw the piece of paper in the trash. When you awake in the morning, make a list of at least three things that you are grateful for. Continue this practice every day and watch your mental and emotional well-being improve.

Notice the Silver Lining

One of the most powerful practices you can adopt is to notice the positive aspects of your life on a regular basis. Begin by looking for the good as often as you can. Perhaps you're driving down the road and you notice that you seem to be catching a lot of green lights—acknowledge it. Maybe you find a quarter on the ground—take note of it. Or you might recognize that your favorite wine is on sale. It really doesn't matter what it is. This practice can be applied to all aspects of life, big or small. And when you notice something positive, do your best to feel the happiness or gratitude in the body for at least 15 seconds. Research has shown this is generally what it takes to encode this information into long-term memory. The goal is to begin to condition your mind, your awareness, into the beautiful aspects of life that are working in your favor. Research has shown that you can change the neural pathways in your brain by putting this into practice, to the point that eventually it can become habit.

Chapter 10

REJUVENATION

I've always said that I will never let an old person into my body.
That is, I don't believe in "thinking" old . . . Don't program yourself
to break down as you age with thoughts that decline is inevitable.

— DR. WAYNE W. DYER

In all the time we spent learning from some of the oldest people around the world, there was one truth that remained blatantly obvious: Father Time bears formidable opposition to our efforts of remaining healthy and youthful. My genuine admiration for Sardinian resident Giulio Podda was profound. To see a 104-year-old man ride a bicycle instantly puts a smile on every onlooker's face. And the astonishment and awe I experienced watching 97-year-old Hideko Kamida till her soil and read the newspaper without glasses will forever live in my memory. Despite the relatively good health and function demonstrated by both Giulio and Hideko, as with all the elders I met, there was a clear recognition of significant cognitive and physical decline that could not be dismissed. After all, it is expected that anyone crossing the threshold of 90 or 100 years would likely have severely diminished hearing, eyesight, and physical mobility. But we are now entering an era where that may not be the continued expectation.

There is no denying it. Humanity is poised for an evolutionary leap in its ability to rejuvenate the human body through the use of regenerative medicine techniques and antiaging therapies. The emergence of regenerative technologies, utilization of biologic agents, and implementation of restorative procedures coupled with the speed at which they are developing is revolutionizing the way we approach damaged tissue and dysfunction.

There is so much to be excited for as the advancements in regenerative medicine continue to make their way into the mainstream and become less expensive, more readily available, and are used with ever-greater proficiency. Without a doubt, what is proving to be most effective and safe in the field of regenerative medicine are therapeutic technologies and methods that mimic nature or directly utilize organic biologic agents. Some of the more promising emergent therapies include the innovative use of light, sound, peptides, hormones, stem cells, and oxygen. Technology is also getting exponentially faster, smaller, and more efficient, allowing for more precise application of these and other therapeutic agents.

Regenerative medicine is still in its infancy, but I suspect that, based on the success rates seen in clinics today around the world, at some point in the not-too-distant future its use will eclipse or categorically replace modern Western medicine. The amazing clinical outcomes seen in regenerative medicine clinics simply cannot be duplicated by traditional medical practices that merely cut away tissue, add artificial structures and supports, chemically attack, or use medications to subvert symptoms. There is no doubt that many of these methods can save lives, but when it comes to their regenerative capacity, they are crude at best. To the contrary, the precision application of biological agents and therapies that mimic nature are reversing the symptoms of autism, putting cancer into remission, reversing type 1 and type 2 diabetes, restoring eyesight, eliminating arthritic pain, restoring joint integrity and mobility, regrowing cartilage and tendons, restoring cardiac function, and reversing neurodegenerative conditions and more. While the therapeutic potential of regenerative medicine is tremendous, it seems negligent to solely rely on these novel therapies as a cure-all for chronic disease and age-related degeneration. Rather, they are best thought of as a corrective therapeutic option and supplemental to a harmonious lifestyle as outlined in the majority of this book.

If you do not live in alignment with your constitution or follow the principles of nature and the demands of your own biology, there is no promise that even the most exciting regenerative therapies on the horizon will do much to extend life by any significant degree. What is most promising, however, is the degree to which the evolving regenerative technologies and antiaging therapies can help us to preserve our youthful function, age more gracefully, and with far less pain and suffering.

STEM CELL THERAPY

Perhaps the most revolutionary and exciting area of regenerative medicine currently involves the use of stem cells to both treat and prevent disease. The reason for this is because stem cells have the unique ability to renew themselves and are the functional cellular building blocks of all bodily tissue. While there are a variety of stem cell types based on specific characteristics, they all carry out three main functions in the body. The first is to reproduce themselves. The second is to differentiate and become new tissue, such as bone, cartilage, liver, or nerve cells, for example. And the third function is to initiate repair of damaged tissue.

According to Dr. Neil Riordan, a leading stem cell expert, the primary benefits of stem cell therapy result not from their ability to become new cell types, but rather from their propensity to secrete molecular messengers that stimulate the growth and repair of damaged cells. As part of this process they also send signals to induce functional changes and influence the behavior of dysfunctional cells. Stem cells even have the ability to donate mitochondria to damaged cells. What's more, stem cells also seem to preferentially move toward and initiate repair in the most damaged cells. Stem cell therapy has been successfully used in the treatment of cancer, autism, coronavirus infections, type 1 and type 2 diabetes, autoimmune diseases, joint deterioration, back issues, neurodegenerative conditions, cardiovascular diseases, and arthritic conditions, to name a few.

As of the time of this writing, the use of stem cells in the United States is quite limited compared with a handful of other countries around the world. And the stem cell treatment industry in the United States is unfortunately still very much operating like the Wild West. There are a variety of different stem cells types and sources, all with their own unique applications and benefits. Currently, the most promising type of stem cells used by the leading clinics around the globe are mesenchymal stem cells (MSCs). These stem cells can be extracted from various bodily tissues including placentas, umbilical cord, amniotic fluid, skin, fat cells, bone marrow, and even menstrual blood. For purposes of prevention and treatment of disease, stem cells extracted from live, healthy birth tissue such as the umbilical cord has demonstrated to be the preferred source of MSCs, as the extraction doesn't require harm to a new life. And due to the rich vitality of young living tissue, these stems cells have proven to be highly potent. Once extracted, these cells can be screened and cultured in a lab using various growth factors. And then they can be injected into any patient as needed. Except for certain cancer therapies and special cases approved by the FDA, this method is not legal in the United States, but it is utilized with great success in many countries around the world.

In the United States, stem cells are typically harvested from the patient's own fat tissue or bone marrow and, with minimal processing, get injected back into the patient the same day. This is known as an autologous stem cell transplant and is often used to treat joint and spinal injuries, among other conditions. One of the primary limitations with this method, however, has to do with the age of the patient and severity of the injury or condition. In older patients, autologous stem cell transplants tend to be less effective because they inherently have fewer stem cells to extract and the quality of the available stem cells tends to diminish the older we get.

When you're young, you have a large pool of healthy, well-functioning stem cells. Over time, cellular damage accumulates, and your pool of healthy stem cells declines at an exponential rate, limiting your ability to regenerate healthy tissue. This is one of the primary reasons young children heal so quickly compared with adults. To quantify the difference in magnitude, researchers placed stem cells from a newborn baby in a laboratory culture medium and found that they will divide approximately every 24 hours. At the end of 30 days, approximately 1 billion stem cells will have proliferated. Stem cells from an average middle-age adult, on the other hand, only divide every 2 days on average, resulting in only about 32,000 stem cells at the end of 30 days. And this decline continues precipitously into old age. This means that the older or less healthy we become, the more advantageous it becomes to use postnatal sources of stem cells instead of our own.

Stem Cell Potency

As the research and practice of stem cell therapy has progressed over the past several years, experts have begun to realize that not all stem cells are created equal. There is research currently being done to identify and select the most effective stem cells with the best molecular signature and most promising healing potential. Dr. Riordan has trademarked these cells "Golden Cells."

Another important factor that determines the potency of stem cell therapy is the how the stem cells are handled and stored after they are extracted from the source. Freezing and thawing stem cells invariably results in a loss of vitality, coherence, and function. As a result, frozen and thawed stem cells must be re-cultured to activate their healing potential. Interestingly, stems cells that are "dead" or that have lost much of their vitality can still have some healing potential, but not to the degree they did prior to being frozen and thawed. Because of this, some researchers are focusing on more effective ways to culture stem cells in the lab using novel growth factors and specific preservation methods that don't involve freezing and thawing. Researchers have also potentially identified ways of enhancing the proliferation and activation of otherwise dormant stem cells using specific frequencies of light, resulting in greater cell signaling and repair of tissue.

There is so much going on in the world of stem cell therapy and in the coming few years, there is poised to be an explosion of uses even beyond what is available today. As we wait for the dust to settle in this industry, there are a few things that remain abundantly clear. And that is that not all stem cells have equal potency and the methods by which stem cells are harvested, processed, and stored have a tremendous impact on the effectiveness and safety of the treatment. Like most industries, technological innovation will continue to drive down cost, increase availability, and improve the effectiveness of stem cell treatment over the next decade. And it should be no surprise to see stem cells become the most widely used treatment for a majority of injuries and diseases because the treatment fundamentally relies on the innate wisdom and intelligence of the most coherent cells in the human body.

REGENERATIVE ORTHOPEDICS

Researchers agree that exercise is one of the most valuable tools to preserve muscle mass, cardiovascular health, and cognitive function as we age. But this becomes easier said than done when you're dealing with debilitating hip pain, arthritic knees, or chronic back issues. Until recently, there just wasn't much in the way of options for real improvement once significant degeneration occurred in musculoskeletal tissues such as ligaments and tendons or spinal discs. Standard arthroscopic procedures require a small incision and the use of a fiber-optic camera to diagnose joint issues and assist in surgery that cuts, shaves, and stitches injured tissue inside the joint. Spinal fusion is still commonplace in an effort to eliminate painful motion of injured and degenerated discs. And nobody wants to replace a joint unless it is the last option. Fortunately, over the past couple decades, the emergent field of regenerative medicine has been increasingly providing real and lasting orthopedic solutions for those suffering from sports injuries as well as degenerative discs and joints. While arthroscopic and joint replacement procedures still serve an invaluable function, there are now less invasive and more effective ways to address many of these acute and degenerative injuries.

Regenerative medicine clinics now have the ability to use a variety of novel procedures that harness the innate intelligence and vitality offered by stem cells, platelet-rich plasma (PRP), and placental matrix and deliver it to musculoskeletal injuries with precision to expedite healing and regrow connective tissues such as ligaments, tendons, cartilage, and fascia.

Platelet-Rich Plasma

The use of platelet-rich plasma has been progressing since the 1970s when it was primarily used in blood transfusions for those who had low platelet count in their blood. Then in the '80s and '90s, it was utilized to enhance wound healing in many dental surgeries, skin grafts, and cosmetic procedures. Now PRP has a wide range of uses to improve healing time and reduce the formation of scar tissue in wound healing. And some of the common uses today include cardiac surgeries, hair regrowth, and to help heal chronic joint pain and spinal disc degeneration.

PRP isn't the most advanced regenerative therapy on the market, but it does serve a valuable role in regenerative medicine, as it can be successfully used to avoid surgery, reduce chronic pain and inflammation, and help restore joint mobility. PRP is also more widely used and affordable than stem cell therapy. And since it makes use of the patient's own blood to heal their injuries, the process of generating PRP is relatively quick and easy. After blood is drawn, it is simply spun down in a matter of minutes such that the platelets and plasma separate from the rest of the blood. This plasma contains a high concentration of platelets that then get injected directly into the injured area right away. This platelet-rich plasma has the capacity to stimulate healing beyond what the aging body would normally be capable of, as it contains a wide variety of growth factors that activate stem cells, modulate inflammation, and encourage tissue remodeling over the course of several weeks after the injection.

Placental Tissue Matrix (PTM) Therapy

In the use of PTM therapy, placental tissue is donated from healthy live births and sterilized before use. This sterilized tissue is injected into the injured region where it has the ability to adhere to damaged tissue. Once in place, the placental tissue delivers a connective collagen matrix that offers anti-inflammatory benefits and supplies a host of extracellular proteins, growth factors, and cytokines that promote endogenous repair mechanisms and work with the body's own cells to modulate healthy tissue reconstruction instead of scar tissue.

Similar to PRP, downtime with this procedure is minimal, usually only a few days. However, the regenerative effects will continue for three to four months before the full benefits are realized.

Nerve Hydrodissection

Nerve hydrodissection is one of the newer methods of treating debilitating chronic pain. In some instances, pain can be caused by nerves that become entrapped or adhere to their surrounding tissue instead of gliding freely. As the nerve gets stretched and compressed through movement, it can cause chronic pain, tingling, or numbness.

The process of nerve hydrodissection requires the use of a needle to inject fluid in the area around the entrapped nerve. The gentle fluid pressure opens the space around the nerve and permanently separates the fascial layers, muscles, or adhesions from the nerve. This allows the nerve to move freely with little friction, improving circulation and creating lasting relief from pain. Nerve hydrodissection is a very quick and safe procedure compared to surgery. Additionally, pain can be resolved almost instantly in some cases and recovery time is minimal, often only a couple weeks. Carpal tunnel is the most commonly treated condition, but nerve hydrodissection is used in regenerative medicine clinics to resolve a variety of peripheral nerve entrapments that lead to chronic pain. Often when pain is eliminated, mobility and range of motion return, which not only improves quality of life but encourages healthy movement into old age.

Ultrasound

One of the most effective and cutting-edge methods used in regenerative medicine is the application of ultrasound to diagnose injuries and evaluate abnormalities in nerves, joints, and connective tissues with much greater detail. It can also be used in the presence of movement to get a better sense for how injured tissue behaves in real-time motion. Because ultrasound is capable of generating such high-resolution images, it can be used to see extremely small structures and abnormalities that would otherwise be missed with MRI technology. Perhaps even more exciting are the novel procedures that use ultrasound to guide regenerative therapeutics such as PRP, placental matrix, or stem cells exactly where the injured tissue requires healing and regeneration. With 10 times the precision of MRI, ultrasound-guided injections result in increased tissue regrowth, faster healing times, and more effective treatments overall.

Ultrasound-guided injections are revolutionizing the treatment of chronic pain and connective tissue injuries. In the coming years, the technology, procedures, and techniques will continue to evolve and improve, as will the skill of the doctors who perform them.

Not every injury or condition offers a straightforward solution. And the decision of whether to use PRP, stem cells, or placental matrix depends on a variety of circumstances that must be evaluated by an experienced doctor with a holistic understanding in order to determine what is optimal for the patient. Like much of the medical profession, or with other skillsets such as cooking or playing the piano, it is in the practitioner's expertise where a lot of variability arises. Working with a skilled practitioner with a lot of experience, good instincts, and gifted precision can make a world of difference with respect to clinical outcomes. Nevertheless, regenerative orthopedics is changing the game when it comes to sports injuries and chronic degenerative discs, joints, and connective tissue.

PEPTIDES

The use of peptides in the world of antiaging and regenerative therapy has exploded the last few years for good reason. Not only have these powerful little molecules been successfully used in the treatment of a wide range of diseases, but they have gained a lot of proponents in the sport of bodybuilding, antiaging clinics, and in regenerative medicine circles for their ability to turn back the biological clock.

Peptides are naturally occurring strings of amino acids that act as endogenous signaling molecules in the body to communicate with cells and tell them how to function. Insulin is one example of the more than 7,000 peptides that are naturally occurring in the human body. And because peptides speak in a language the body understands, it is a therapy that has proven to be extremely safe and effective. Perhaps not surprisingly, we naturally have an abundance of peptides in our youth and levels eventually decline with age.

Each peptide tends to be highly specific in how it works—like having the right set of instructions to carry out very precise epigenetic functions. With this in mind, they can be used in a targeted manner to address a particular health condition by influencing specific biological pathways responsible for improved function or regeneration of a given cell type or even across a wide variety of cell types.

Research has demonstrated that peptides can be used to increase muscle mass, decrease body fat, improve brain function, enhance libido, improve sleep, regrow hair, increase metabolic health, improve gut function, expedite healing, and reduce inflammation, among other things. Because peptides are naturally occurring molecules, they are quite safe to use and difficult to patent. Despite their health-promoting effects and excellent safety profile, most peptides are still not approved by the FDA. Currently, they are still viewed as experimental and are therefore largely unregulated. However, their use has only increased in the past few years as peptide research has developed, and consumers continue to benefit from their profound health-promoting effects.

Most peptides are best taken as injectables because the bioavailability is guaranteed to be near 100 percent. Due to the large size of most peptides, they cannot survive the digestive tract if taken orally, preventing them from reaching the blood stream and ultimately cellular receptor sites. Researchers have identified a few peptides that do have some bioavailability when taken orally and sublingually, and others that are partially absorbed through the skin, but it is unclear just how bioavailable they are compared with subcutaneous injection. So even though peptides are unlikely to be patented directly, there is a lot of intense research attempting to figure out how to make peptides orally bioavailable. This is a significant indication of the huge potential that peptides hold when it comes to improving health and longevity. So while the consumer market for peptides is still in its infancy, this is a therapeutic approach to rejuvenation that is poised to explode over the coming years. What follows are a few notable peptides that are drawing a lot of interest for their potential to accelerate healing, restore function, and regenerate tissue.

BPC-157

BPC is an acronym for a peptide that was discovered and isolated from human stomach acid. They named this peptide "body protective compound" after noticing that the body naturally produces a lot of this peptide as a part of the healing response. BPC-157 is a smaller derivative of the larger BPC protein while still containing many of the healing properties. Numerous animal studies have demonstrated that BPC-157 accelerates healing of the GI tract, muscle, tendons, ligaments, and skin. It also encourages new blood vessel growth, increases growth factors, and reduces oxidative stress. For its wide-ranging benefits and ability to be taken orally, BPC-157 has become one of the most popularly used peptides by regenerative medicine practitioners and biohackers alike.

Thymosin Beta 4

Thymosin Beta 4 (TB4) is a peptide that was first isolated from bovine thymus tissue 40 years ago. While it is present in most human tissues, it is heavily concentrated in the thymus and other lymphoid tissues. Whenever your body experiences injury, TB4 gets secreted. But as your body ages, your ability to produce this healing peptide declines.

Thymosin Beta 4 serves a variety of physiological functions, perhaps most notably to preserve cardiac function and improve cardiovascular health due to its ability to dramatically increase actin, a key cell-building protein. Actin increases blood vessel formation, promotes wound healing, and decreases chronic inflammation. Because heart disease remains one of the primary causes of death in the United States and in many Western countries, TB4 can be of great benefit. Additionally, TB4 helps get wound-healing cells to the sites of injury, which is a big deal since many of them die before reaching their destination. TB4 has also been shown to promote bone remodeling after fractures, increase collagen deposition, accelerate healing of the skin and gut, minimize scar formation, improve immune function, accelerate muscle repair, and improve neurodegenerative conditions.

There is now a derivative of TB4 that has been developed for oral administration called TB4-Frag. Some researchers suggest the oral bioavailability is as high as 90 percent, but this is not yet a consensus view. However, anecdotal information from many integrative practitioners, regenerative medicine experts, and consumers suggest that TB4-Frag has considerable therapeutic value when taken orally.

Epitalon

Epitalon peptide was discovered by Russian scientist Vladimir Khavinson, who performed animal research with it for decades. One of the primary benefits he found was that epitalon promotes the natural production of telomerase, the enzyme responsible for extending telomeres that protect the ends of DNA strands. As we age and cellular coherence is lost, telomerase activity declines, resulting in a more unstable genome and less efficient regeneration. Epitalon has the power to help the body regrow telomeres to maintain a more stable genome. Epitalon has also been shown to increase melatonin production, improve circadian rhythm, regulate immune function, activate growth factors in connective tissue, improve skin health, and decrease tumor growth, among other results.

KPV

KPV is a standout peptide when it comes to reducing intestinal inflammation and improving inflammatory bowel disease (IBD). Discovered in the 1980s, KPV produces its anti-inflammatory effect by downregulating inflammatory cascades inside the cell. Interestingly, KPV becomes even more effective in the presence of IBD because the transport protein that helps KPV get into colon cells is more prevalent in the cases of IBD, Crohn's disease, and ulcerative colitis. As is often the case for therapeutic agents that improve gastrointestinal health, KPV has also been shown to potentially improve chronic inflammatory skin conditions such as psoriasis, eczema, and dermatitis. KPV is another peptide that has good oral bioavailability, and research has demonstrated its effectiveness through oral administration.

At this point, there are dozens of health-promoting peptides that have been discovered and made available to consumers for "research purposes only." While peptides haven't been cleared by the FDA for treatment of disease, this hasn't prevented therapeutic use by regenerative medicine practitioners, biohackers, body builders, and those seeking a cure for their chronic ailments. And it is not uncommon to hear raving reviews from those who have experience and understanding of how to properly use peptides to accelerate healing and improve regeneration.

MELATONIN

Perhaps the most controversial biological molecule in the realm of health and longevity, melatonin is primarily known as the hormone of darkness for its well-established role in helping to regulate the sleep-wake cycle. But the physiological role of melatonin goes far beyond regulating sleep. Melatonin has been shown to correct circadian rhythm disruption, improve mitochondrial function, protect against cancer, improve skin and gut health, reduce chronic inflammation, improve metabolic syndromes, eliminate infection, improve cardiovascular health, increase hair growth, regulate immune function, and improve neurological diseases such as dementia, ALS, MS, and Parkinson's.

There are some health professionals that firmly believe it is not wise to supplement with melatonin, except in extreme cases of insomnia or perhaps to help reset circadian rhythm in the case of jet lag. Other experts believe that supplementing with very low-dose melatonin (less than one milligram) in the evening is a good strategy for most adults. And still other experts prefer doses in the three- to five-milligram range long-term for antiaging benefits. There is another perspective, however, that raises many eyebrows in the medical and scientific community. Researchers and practitioners in this camp believe that supplementing with extreme doses of melatonin in the range of 20 to 400 milligrams per day can be a useful way to combat chronic illness, restore healthy function, and improve longevity.

The research detailing the health-promoting effects of melatonin is vast, using a variety of doses with minimal downsides. And this is what makes melatonin so controversial. The benefits of supplementing with melatonin have been documented using as little as tenths of milligrams per day up to a few hundred milligrams per day for years without any notable side effects. One experiment administered 6.6 grams—that's 6,660 milligrams of melatonin per day to humans for a month without any notable side effects.

LD50 is an established measurement used to quantify the toxicity level of a compound. It is an abbreviation for the average amount of a substance sufficient to kill 50 percent of the population. As an example, the LD50 of table salt is 3 milligrams per kilogram of body weight for a rat. For sugar, the LD50 is 30 grams per kilogram for a rat When it comes to melatonin, researchers have been unable to identify an LD50 for rodents or humans. That's how safe it is. And finding something this safe is particularly strange when it comes to the world of hormones. This is where another wrinkle comes into play. While melatonin is typically classified as a neurohormone, it has some unique aspects that differ from typical hormones—namely that it doesn't require a releasing factor like typical hormones; it is produced in a myriad of tissues throughout the body; melatonin receptors and binding sites are found in just about every cell of the body; and there is no negative feedback loop when one takes supplemental melatonin. Your pineal won't shut down production of melatonin because it is fundamentally controlled by light through the eyes and, to a lesser degree, on the skin. So it appears that no matter how much melatonin you might take, your body will not shut down its endogenous production or alter its tolerance.

Evidence suggests that melatonin is both taken up by mitochondria and also likely to be produced inside mitochondria. This means that every cell of your body is making and utilizing melatonin except red blood cells. As such, it serves a huge role in protecting mitochondria, DNA, and cellular architecture. Research has found that oocytes—female germ cells that will eventually become eggs—synthesize large amounts of melatonin during maturation, which helps them increase mitochondrial DNA, produce more energy, reduce oxidative stress, and protect against DNA mutation from oxidative stress. The ability for your body to make new, healthy mitochondria is also regulated by melatonin. And it has been found to promote mitophagy, the recycling and clearing of old, damaged mitochondria, which helps to improve cellular energetics and reduce cellular damage. When mitochondria fail to make adequate melatonin, this loss invariably results in greater cellular degeneration and DNA damage.

Melatonin is present in just about all bodily fluids as well, including cerebrospinal fluid, saliva, bile, synovial fluid, amniotic fluid, and breast milk. And in some of these fluids, melatonin levels exceed concentrations measured in the blood. What's more, virtually all the microbes in your gastrointestinal tract also respond to and utilize melatonin. The ubiquitous use of melatonin throughout the body helps explain the myriad of effects demonstrated by research studies throughout the decades.

Melatonin and Inflammation

There are three primary mechanisms through which a molecule is able to defend against free-radical damage in the body. One is by scavenging free radicals directly through a molecule's electrical and structural composition. Think of this like soldiers on the front line. In this way, the damaging free radical is neutralized by an antioxidant molecule. Melatonin is unique in that it does not promote oxidation under any circumstance, and it produces metabolites that also act as antioxidants.

The second method of reducing oxidative damage occurs when a molecule is capable of stimulating antioxidant enzymes that act as a defense against inflammatory free radicals. This would be like a military general who sends specific soldiers and battalions to the front line of war as needed.

The third method involves a molecule that is capable of directly inhibiting free radical enzymes from expressing. This would be like someone stealing the weaponry of the enemy, so they have no way to do damage. Interestingly, melatonin has all three antioxidant capabilities. It is an extremely powerful antioxidant, capable of directly mopping up excess inflammation. It has the capacity to signal the production of superoxide dismutase, catalase, and glutathione—all three of which are powerful cellular antioxidant enzymes. And lastly, melatonin can also downregulate the expression of the proinflammatory enzyme known as inducible nitric oxide synthase.

With these effects in mind, extremely high doses of supplemental melatonin makes sense to help resolve chronic inflammatory conditions. One study demonstrated that 300 milligrams of melatonin taken rectally for up to two years proved to be safe and effective for reducing elevated oxidative stress in ALS patients back down to levels typically seen in the average population.

My own personal experience taking 200 to 300 milligrams of melatonin daily resulted in a marked reduction in inflammatory lab markers as well as softer skin with less dryness, improved muscle and joint pain, and better stool formation. It only took about a week or so to start noticing improvements and I continued taking a couple hundred milligrams almost daily for months. I never had any issues with sleep and noticed no downside effects. Similar results have been experienced by my clients as well. I noticed lab values of the oxidative stress marker 8-OHdG, one of the best markers to estimate DNA damage, consistently decrease and chronic symptoms improve or completely resolve on a very regular basis.

Melatonin and Gut

One of the lesser-known aspects of melatonin physiology is that the human gastrointestinal tract contains 400 times more melatonin than does the pineal gland. The release of gastrointestinal melatonin has less to do with light and more to do with food intake and extended fasting, both of which seem to upregulate GI melatonin levels. Research demonstrates that the microbes in your gut are heavily influenced by circadian rhythm and melatonin fluctuations—perhaps unsurprisingly, since these microbes are constantly receiving signals from the entire body. What may be surprising is that melatonin plays a massive role in the composition, diversity, and the rhythmic alterations of gut microbiota.

Mental/emotional stress and sleep deprivation negatively impact microbiota populations, resulting in decreased diversity and elevated levels of GI inflammation. Fortunately, exogenous melatonin treatment has been shown to attenuate the harmful effects of stress and sleep deprivation, as it increases the population of a number of commensal (beneficial) microbes in the GI tract. Some of the microbes identified include Akkermansia muciniphila, Lactobacillus, Enterobacter aerogenes, and Faecalibacterium prausnitzii, which collectively have been shown to reduce GI inflammation, lower body weight, heal fatty liver disease, and improve insulin resistance. Evidence continues to mount that the population and behavior of many, if not most commensal gut microbes may be highly sensitive to fluctuating melatonin levels. If so, the implications of improving gut health with exogenous melatonin are profound.

There is another aspect of GI health that melatonin impacts as well. It helps tonify or strengthen the parasympathetic nervous system, which enervates the entire gastrointestinal tract. Thanks to modern technology, parasympathetic tone can now easily be tracked by measuring heart rate variability. Good parasympathetic tone is absolutely necessary for proper digestion and detoxification, among other things. More directly, melatonin impacts the GI tract by improving the health of the mucosal lining and helping to regenerate the intestinal epithelium, both of which are critical aspects of healing leaky gut and eliminating food sensitivities that have become so common.

Melatonin and Immune Function

Even in healthy aging, immune function begins to deteriorate well before midlife. That's because, in part, the thymus gland reaches peak size and function in adolescence and then begins to age faster than most other organs. The thymus is one of the body's primary immune organs. Not only does it play a central role in the development of T-cells, it also produces inflammatory cytokines, interleukins, hormones, and peptides that are all essential to a balanced immune response and proper inflammatory regulation. While researchers have yet to elucidate a full picture, it is clear that the thymus plays an important role in regulating neuroendocrine hormonal function as well.

As the thymus begins to atrophy in our early teens, healthy tissue is progressively replaced by adipose tissue throughout life. The peak decline in thymic weight starts to occur around age 35. And by age 40, only 30 percent of thymic weight and function typically remains. At age 75, the thymus is only operating around 20 percent of what it did in our early teens. Age-related thymic decline can result in greater susceptibility to infection, an increase in food sensitivities, autoimmunity, poor blood sugar control, systemic inflammation, and a loss of coherence in the neuroendocrine hormonal network.

Dr. Walter Pierpaoli is one of the world's leading anti-aging and longevity researchers. His research on melatonin has demonstrated a profound link between the pineal gland and the thymus. In one experiment, Dr. Pierpaoli's team switched the pineal glands in old mice and young mice. This pineal cross-transplantation resulted in the young mice with old pineal glands aging rapidly, showing all the hallmarks of old age, including cataracts and muscle wasting. And the old mice with young pineal glands regained vitality, showed increased muscle mass, and regrew healthy coats. Autopsies revealed significant degeneration of the thymus glands in the young mice with old pineal glands. Meanwhile the old mice with young pineal glands saw their thymus regenerate. This and other follow-up experiments have confirmed a definitive bidirectional link between the thymus, the pineal gland, and its primary hormone, melatonin.

In line with Dr. Pierpaoli's experiments, supplementing with exogenous melatonin has been shown to effectively help to regrow thymus tissue and restore thymus cell function in age-related decline. Along with melatonin, zinc is an important co-factor in helping to restore integrity and intelligence of thymus tissue.

Melatonin can also play a powerful role in mitigating symptoms of autoimmune disease. In fact, research has shown that supplementing with exogenous melatonin can have a beneficial effect on type 1 diabetes, lupus, and multiple sclerosis. And the mechanisms appear fairly straightforward. T-helper cells known as Th1 and Th17 serve a proinflammatory role in the body. While both are a necessary part of the immune system, they can be a major driver of autoimmune symptoms when they chronically overexpress. Studies show that exogenous melatonin supplementation can decrease Th1 and Th17 expression while increasing the expression of regulatory T-cell function and anti-inflammatory immune signals, major pieces of the puzzle to regain self-tolerance and resolve autoimmune symptoms.

Melatonin and Aging Hormones

Through studies done by researchers like Dr. Pierpaoli and others, it has been established that there is a complex hormonal interplay between the pineal gland, hypothalamus, pituitary, and thymus. In particular, melatonin seems to have a complex regulatory effect on luteinizing hormone (LH), follicle-stimulating hormone (FSH), growth hormone, cortisol, DHEA, testosterone, and estrogen. Of these hormones, there are two that stand out when it comes to the interplay between melatonin and aging. These are luteinizing hormone and follicle-stimulating hormone. At the onset of puberty, boys and girls both experience a sharp and sustained drop in melatonin levels, followed by dramatic rise in LH and FSH, triggering sexual development in both boys and girls. And data on children who experience a significant delay in puberty, medically termed *constitutional delayed puberty,* show that they have significantly elevated melatonin levels and low LH and FSH. So there is a meaningful and causal inverse relationship between levels of melatonin and levels of LH and FSH. It appears that melatonin acts as a brake for rising LH and FSH levels.

In aging adults, there is a similar phenomenon that occurs over the span of 30-plus years as opposed to the sudden shift at the onset of puberty. Peak nighttime melatonin levels decline about 70 percent from ages 25 to age 50 in both men and women. Meanwhile, from about 50 to 55 years old and onward, LH and FSH levels rise considerably. For women, these shifts accelerate at the onset of menopause. These hormonal shifts have prompted researchers to suspect that melatonin levels may play some regulatory role in the onset of menopause. While the mechanisms are still unsettled, studies and anecdotal reports have shown that supplementing with as little as three milligrams of melatonin at night can delay and in some cases reverse menopause in women. In these studies, perimenopausal and menopausal women reported less depression and general improvement in mood as well. Melatonin supplementation has also been shown to prevent post-menopausal bone loss. Based on the research, women over 60 years old may benefit from taking more than three milligrams of melatonin in order to elicit similar effects. Unfortunately, there is a serious lack of research investigating higher doses in elderly women.

Hormones are powerful signaling molecules that have wide-ranging epigenetic implications throughout the body. Evidence suggests that by maintaining more youthful levels of hormones such as melatonin, LH, and FSH, you can maintain more youthful epigenetic expression and function as you age. It is worth noting that when fasting from food, melatonin tends to increase while LH and FSH decline—yet another instance that shows the inverse relationship between these hormones and another benefit of fasting.

Melatonin, Pregnancy, and Birth Control

One of the more fascinating aspects of melatonin is its ability to increase likelihood of pregnancy as well as its use as a female contraceptive. Melatonin helps reduce excessive oxidative stress, and thus damage to DNA, mitochondria, and cell membranes. For this reason, it has been shown to increase the health of oocytes (immature egg cells) in women as well as the health of sperm cells in men. Additionally, it also improves the health of endometrial tissues in women and balance hormonal profiles of women with PCOS and menstrual irregularity. Research on in-vitro fertilization has demonstrated that three milligrams of melatonin taken nightly from day five of a woman's menstrual cycle onward, can successfully increase fertilization rates and result in healthier embryos overall.

When it comes to contraception, melatonin has also been used along with exogenous progesterone to reduce likelihood of pregnancy. Research has shown that high-dose melatonin in the range of 75 milligrams to 300 milligrams plus progesterone can be used as an effective form of oral contraceptive. This study lasted four months and not only were no side effects of any kind reported, but the combination of melatonin and progesterone did not disrupt sleep-wake rhythms in any of the women. An additional study used 75 milligrams of melatonin for as long as three years without any negative side effects.

Melatonin Dosing

From my personal experience as a user and as a practitioner, there is a wide range of uses for melatonin. And finding the right dose for each individual is a matter of trial and a little educated guessing, mostly because there hasn't been enough research done to find optimal doses in a variety of circumstances. There are a few things to consider when supplementing with melatonin. First are the three primary routes of administration—orally, liposomal delivery, and suppository. Unfortunately, the bioavailability of standard oral administration is anywhere from 1 to 74 percent, according to research. For this reason, liposomal delivery and suppository forms offer the best absorption and bioavailability. Another important factor to generate positive results is to keep your plasma levels of melatonin elevated for extended periods of time. To get maximum advantage of melatonin's night-time benefits, sustained release works best.

For children with sleep disorders, ADHD, or symptoms of autism, 3 milligrams to 10 milligrams has been successfully used in studies without side effects. However, for most children with neurological disorders, developmental challenges, autism, and sleep disorders, it is prudent to start at a low dosage of 0.3 milligrams and increase every two to four weeks as needed. An effective and optimal dose may be found at levels below 3 milligrams.

For adults with insomnia, research shows that 75 milligrams of melatonin per night results in an increase in total sleep time at night and alertness during the day.

Most adults between the ages of 30 to 65 who want to mitigate minor symptoms or general age-related decline, may find it worthwhile to explore doses ranging from 10 to 100 milligrams per night ongoing until symptoms subside. In my experience, most people start to notice positive changes after two to three weeks of nightly supplementation at a sufficient dosage. While most can tolerate high levels of melatonin right away and there is little risk of taking too much, some may prefer a gradual increase. Therefore, it may be beneficial to start at 10 milligrams per night and double the dose every two weeks until you reach a dose that feels comfortable for you.

For those suffering from chronic fatigue, chronic gastrointestinal symptoms, chronic skin conditions, food sensitivities, mold infections, Lyme disease, and otherwise unknown complex chronic illness, doses ranging from 10 milligrams per night up to 400 milligrams may be helpful. Again, starting low and doubling every two weeks is an effective approach. Across many chronic ailments, typical improvements include softer and more even-colored skin, improved bowel regularity, better sleep, better mood, reduced chronic pain, decreased inflammation, and improved cognitive function.

In elderly adults, doses as low as 0.3 milligram have been shown to mimic nighttime physiological levels of younger adults. This may be all that is required to improve age-related sleep decline. However, there may be more to be gained by increasing the dose, particularly when it comes to preventing neurodegeneration. High-dose melatonin has been shown to be neuroprotective by reducing oxidative damage, modulating inflammatory cascades, and increasing neurotrophins like brain-derived neurotrophic factor and nerve growth factor, which promote the survival and growth of new brain cells. Additionally, the aging brain tends to accumulate beta-amyloid, tao protein, and alpha-synuclein, proteins associated with elevated brain inflammation. The glymphatic system, which is primarily activated during deep sleep, is responsible for clearing out these proteins along with other waste. Using melatonin can help improve parasympathetic tone and increase deep sleep, thus improving glymphatic clearance, quelling brain inflammation, and preventing protein accumulation over time.

Melatonin has been studied and used in the treatment of a wide variety of cancers, both independently as well as in combination with chemotherapy and other medications. The results have proven positive at a wide variety of doses. In the case of cancer, it is best to work with an integrative cancer doctor to determine the appropriate dosage and application.

Studies have shown that for those with liver damage, the metabolization of melatonin may be quite delayed, resulting in slower onset and clearance. To compensate for this delay, melatonin can be taken two to four hours before bed so as not to be groggy the following day.

When it comes to melatonin, finding the appropriate or optimal dosage for each individual is perhaps the biggest unknown. However, the level of caution generated by doctors, health practitioners, and the general public appears to be greatly overstated and has no basis in scientific research whatsoever. The therapeutic potential that melatonin holds is quite remarkable given its over-the-counter status and ubiquitous nature in the marketplace. To think of melatonin as merely a sleeping aid is to radically underestimate the myriad of benefits it can exert by reducing inflammation throughout your body and encouraging greater coherence at the level of the gut microbiota, mitochondria, and DNA.

BEYOND LONGEVITY

We currently stand at the forefront of the most dramatic acceleration of health-related technological innovation in recorded history. The most promising therapies over the next 10 to 20 years include the precision use of biological agents that harness the human body's innate wisdom to increase vitality, communication, and coherence between mitochondria, microbiota, and DNA across multiple tissues and systems throughout the individual. Currently, the most promising biological agents include peptides, hormones, stem cells, and other postnatal tissues. But as research continues and new applications develop, there are sure to be new biological agents that emerge and prove useful as regenerative therapies.

There is yet another classification of health technology that shows tremendous potential and is worth plenty of excitement. This class includes devices that utilize sound, light, electricity, magnetism, and oxygen to revitalize the body and increase coherence. There are dozens of effective tools on the market today that use low level lasers, LED lights, pulsed electromagnetic fields (PEMF), electrical stimulation, magnetism, sound waves, ozone, hyperbaric oxygen, and more. Depending on the condition, any number of these technologies may be useful. Innovation in health technology over the past 20 years in particular has brought with it a democratization and decentralization of medical treatment. Access to a hospital or clinic is not required to benefit from these emerging technologies, some of which only cost a couple hundred dollars. The retail market for high-tech health equipment is showing no signs of slowing down. And as health data becomes more available through wearable devices, the patient is more likely to become their own doctor.

The utility of medical technology and regenerative therapies is hard to understate. And yet the old adage cannot be discarded: "An ounce of prevention is worth a pound of cure." Technology cannot compensate for a life lived in ill health. While physical, mental, and emotional health in old age are to be cherished, there is more to life than the pursuit of longevity. Health and disease alike can be wonderful guides on a path toward greater truth and realization that unveils itself by living from the heart in true alignment.

INDEX

D

ABOUT THE AUTHOR

Jason Prall is a former mechanical engineer turned educator, health practitioner, speaker, and filmmaker. Due to 20 years of his own health challenges, Jason discovered the reality behind his symptoms. Through this process, he began working remotely with individuals around the world to provide solutions for those suffering from complex health issues that their doctors were unable to resolve. In 2016, Jason transitioned from working in the integrative disease-care model to a model of health optimization and lifestyle medicine. These lessons culminated in the documentary film series *The Human Longevity Project*, which uncovers the complex mechanisms of chronic disease and aging and the true nature of longevity in our modern world. You can visit him online at beyondlongevitybook.com.

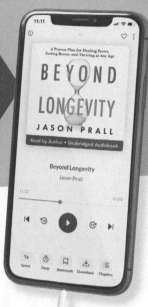